ANNUAL REVIEW OF NURSING RESEARCH

Volume 14, 1996

ANNUAL REVIEW OF NURSING RESEARCH

Volume 14, 1996

Joyce J. Fitzpatrick, Ph.D.
Jane Norbeck, D.N.Sc.

Editors

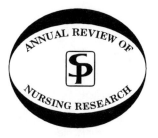

SPRINGER PUBLISHING COMPANY
New York

Order ANNUAL REVIEW OF NURSING RESEARCH. Volume 15, 1997, prior to publication and receive a 10% discount. An order coupon can be found at the back of this volume.

Springer Publishing Company, Inc.
536 Broadway
New York, NY 10012

96 97 98 99 00 / 5 4 3 2 1

ISBN-0-8261-8233-X
ISSN-0739-6686

ANNUAL REVIEW OF NURSING RESEARCH is indexed in *Cumulative Index to Nursing and Allied Health Literature and Index Medicus.*

Printed in the United States of America

Contents

Preface

The *Annual Review of Nursing Research* series is now a well-established part of the scientific literature in nursing. As the series has developed, we have witnessed a narrowing of chapter topics consistent with the expansion of nursing research. Volume 14 reflects this scientific development.

In Part I, Research on Nursing Practice, five chapters focused on nursing interventions are included. Sue A. Thomas and Freda DeKeyser present research on blood pressure. Nancy McCain and Janice Zeller review research on psychoneuroimmunological studies in HIV disease. Delirium intervention research in acute care settings is reviewed by Diane Cronin-Stubbs. Mary Ellen Wewers and Karen Ahijevych present smoking-cessation interventions in chronic illness, and Carol Smith reviews research on quality of life and caregiving in technological home care.

Part II, Nursing Care Delivery, includes two chapters. Gail Ingersoll describes organizational redesign and Barbara Mark presents research on organizational culture.

Part III and Part IV include one chapter each. In the Nursing Education section, Linda Workman reviews oncology education research, and in the section on the profession of nursing, Virginia Cassidy presents research on moral competency.

We are pleased to include two international chapters in this volume. Hava Golander and Tamar Krulik review nursing research in Israel and Isabel Mendes and Maria Trevizan review nursing research in Brazil. We look forward to extending our international efforts in future volumes.

JOYCE J. FITZPATRICK
SENIOR EDITOR

vii

Contributors

Karen L. Ahijevych, PhD
College of Nursing
The Ohio State University
Columbus, OH

Virginia R. Cassidy, EdD
School of Nursing
Northern Illinois University
DeKalb, IL

Diane Cronin-Stubbs, PhD
College of Nursing
Rush University
Chicago, IL

Freda DeKeyser, PhD
School of Nursing
Hadassah Hospital/Hebrew
   University
Jerusalem, ISRAEL

Hava Golander, PhD
Department of Nursing
Tel Aviv University
Ramat Aviv, ISRAEL

Gail L. Ingersoll, EdD
School of Nursing
Indiana University
Indianapolis, IN

Tamar Krulik, DNSc
Department of Nursing
Tel Aviv University
Ramat Aviv, ISRAEL

Barbara A. Mark, PhD
School of Nursing
Medical College of Virginia
Virginia Commonwealth University
Richmond, VA

Nancy L. McCain, DSN
School of Nursing
Virginia Commonwealth University
Richmond, VA

Isabel Amélia Costa Mendes, PhD
College of Nursing
University of São Paulo
   at Ribeirão Preto
Ribeirão Preto, BRAZIL

Carol E. Smith, PhD
School of Nursing
University of Kansas
Kansas City, KS

Sue A. Thomas, PhD
Siegel and Thomas Healthcare Group
Ellicott City, MD

Maria Auxiliadora Trevizan, PhD
College of Nursing
University of São Paulo
   at Ribeirão Preto
Ribeirão Preto, BRAZIL

Mary Ellen Wewers, PhD
College of Nursing
The Ohio State University
Columbus, OH

M. Linda Workman, PhD
Frances Payne Bolton School
   of Nursing
Case Western Reserve University
Cleveland, OH

Janice M. Zeller, PhD
College of Nursing
Rush University
Chicago, IL

Forthcoming

ANNUAL REVIEW OF
NURSING RESEARCH, Volume 15

Tentative Contents

PART I

Research on Nursing Practice

Chapter 1

Blood Pressure

SUE A. THOMAS
SIEGEL AND THOMAS HEALTHCARE GROUP
ELLICOTT CITY, MD

FREDA DEKEYSER
SCHOOL OF NURSING
HADASSAH HOSPITAL/HEBREW UNIVERSITY

CONTENTS

William Harvey, in 1628, was the first to describe the heart and circulation (Willius & Keys, 1941). However, it was not until 1904 that N. S. Korotokov developed the technique to measure blood pressure (BP) noninvasively in humans (Geddis, Hoff, & Badger, 1967). Today BP is one of the most common measurements used to evaluate the cardiovascular system. The most serious physiological consequence of elevated BP is the development of essential hypertension.

Hypertension is a multifactorial psychophysiological disorder. Multiple physiological, behavioral, psychological, and social factors influence BP and contribute to the development of hypertension.

Although nursing is frequently referred to as a biopsychosocial discipline, research in "social" or sociological factors in BP has been neglected (Thomas, Liehr, DeKeyser, & Friedmann, 1993). Scientists in other fields have investigated the effect on BP of social factors such as race and social status. Although race has major biological components, sociological influences also can have profound effects. The research from other disciplines on these factors is reviewed briefly.

SOCIAL FACTORS

Race

Mild to moderate hypertension is 1.5 to 2 times greater for African Americans than for Whites, and severe hypertension is 5 to 7 times more prevalent in African Americans in the United States (Saunders, 1991). African American women have 4½ times higher incidence of hypertension than Caucasian women (American Heart Association, 1992). There are several hypotheses to explain these differences. First, there are several physiological differences that affect BP in these groups, including genetics, sodium excretion, renin-kallikrein-kinin system, potassium intake, and sympathetic nervous system levels (Saunders, 1991). Second, there are several sociological differences, including socioeconomic status (SES), income, and education, each of which is inversely related to the prevalence of hypertension (Calhoun, 1992; Saunders, 1991). Third, researchers have postulated that the combination of increased reactivity to stress in African Americans (Light, Obrist, Sherwood, James, & Strogatz, 1987) and increased environmental stress lead to earlier cardiovascular damage and hypertension (Calhoun, 1992).

Social Status

Distinctions between the effects of race versus social status on BP are hard to define when discussing African Americans. Many studies have shown interaction effects between race and social status on BP. When Klag and co-workers (Klag, Whelton, Coresh, Grim, & Kuller, 1991) tried to determine the relationship between skin color and BP, they found that systolic blood pressure (SBP) and diastolic blood pressure (DBP) were higher in darker persons and increased by 2 mm Hg for every 1 SD increase in skin darkness. However, this association was found only in those with lower SES. The authors postulated that this association may have been due to either a lower ability of those of lower SES to deal with the psychosocial stresses related to darker skin color or an interaction between SES and a susceptible gene that has a higher prevalence in those with darker skin color.

Dressler (1990) tried to determine a possible explanation for the inverse relationship between education and BP. In a study of African Americans, Dressler found that the degree of lifestyle incongruity (defined as the degree to which accumulation of consumer goods and exposure to mass media exceeded the level of education) was associated with higher SBP and DBP. In an effort to sort out the effects of race and social status on African Americans, Fumo and co-workers (1992) evaluated differences in ambulatory blood pressure monitor (ABPM) readings between U.S. Whites, African Americans, and South African Blacks. No differences were found in the daytime BPs. However, African Americans' BPs did not fall as much as did those of the other two groups at night. The authors concluded that the differences in BP between U.S. Whites and African Americans are environmental rather than racial in origin.

Perceived social status also has been shown to affect BP measurements. Reiser and co-workers (Reiser, Reeves, & Armington, 1958) found that army recruits had higher BPs when they were measured by a captain versus a private. Others (Long, Lynch, Machiran, Thomas, & Malinow, 1982) found that BPs were higher when the subject perceived that he/she was talking to a person of higher status. A corollary of social status is the phenomenon called "white coat hypertension." It has been shown that a subset of patients have higher BPs when measured by a physician, compared to those measured by a nurse or a technician or when BP was measured at home. Some have estimated that as many as 20% to 38% of patients experience this phenomenon (Pickering & James, 1989).

The view of BP has expanded from a purely physiological indicator of internal cardiovascular functioning to include the psychosocial aspects of BP. This type of research has many direct clinical applications. For example, if the subset of patients who display white-coat hypertension could be identified, then those patients could have their BP monitored by nurses or technicians.

SCOPE OF THIS REVIEW

Nursing research using BP as an outcome variable has increased in the past decade (Thomas et al., 1993). This review examines nursing BP research from a biopsychosocial perspective. Research by nurses using BP as an outcome variable is identified, described, and discussed. Recommendations for future research also are presented. To identify studies in which BP was used as an outcome variable, a computerized search of MEDLINE and Cumulative Index to Nursing and Allied Health Literature (CINHAL) data bases for the years 1983 through 1993 was done, utilizing the term *blood pressure* as the key word. The search was limited to sources published in readily available journals at two university health science libraries. Abstracts; review articles; studies of infants, children, and adolescents; and articles published in obscure journals were excluded. In addition, when an author was found who had published two or more studies, a search using that author's name was conducted, to ensure a comprehensive review of that nurse's research.

This review of nursing literature begins with a discussion of 7 articles related to measurement issues and reviews 56 nursing studies.

MEASUREMENT OF BLOOD PRESSURE

Advances in the technology to measure BP and in methodology of BP measurement was the focus of seven studies.

Chyun (1985) found that auscultatory SBP and DBP readings were higher than intraarterial readings in cardiac surgery patients, but only the DBP readings were statistically different. Others (Rebenson-Piano, Holm, Foreman, & Kirchhoff, 1989) found that in normotensive and hypertensive intensive care unit (ICU) patients, automated and auscultatory SBP readings were significantly lower than intraarterial measurements. Byra-Cook, Dracup, and Lazik (1990) compared direct BP readings to indirect readings, using different parts of the stethoscope (the bell vs. the diaphragm) and different auscultatory sites (antecubital fossa and 2 cm above on the upper arm). Correlations between direct and indirect SBP and DBP readings were found to be highly correlated ($r > .8$) with both the bell and the diaphragm and at both sites. Indirect readings using the bell/antecubital fossa technique were most accurate when comparing direct and indirect systolic pressures. Indirect readings using the diaphragm/antecubital fossa technique were most accurate when comparing direct and indirect diastolic pressures.

Direct and indirect BP measurements are comparable but not identical because of inherent physiological, instrumentation, and methodological differences in the two techniques (Rebenson-Piano, Holm, & Powers, 1987). Researchers who have compared these two methods have shown that indirect methods may underestimate SBP and overestimate DBP when compared to intraarterial measures (Rebenson-Piano et al., 1987). The preferred measurement technique depends on many factors. The researcher must choose the technique that best fits the requirements of the research.

Three researchers evaluated the best technique for auscultatory BP readings. Mauro (1988) determined that the mean systolic value is greater when measured with the bell as opposed to the diaphragm portion of the stethoscope, whereas the bell decreases the fifth-phase diastolic value. Tachovsky (1985) found that SBP was lower and DBP was higher at the forearm as opposed to the upper arm in nonobese women. Significant differences between auscultatory SBP readings in the right and left arms also were found, but these differences were not attributable to size of arterial diameter (Biddle & Te, 1986). Research on methodology of measurement of BP is an important area of nursing research. The use of the traditional site of measurement (upper arm), use of bell, and differences in arms have been confirmed as valid.

Ambulatory Blood Pressure Monitoring

Blood pressure is a dynamic physiological parameter and can vary from minute to minute. The most common indirect method of measurement of BP is made by a sphygmomanometer and a stethoscope. This method has several disadvantages. One of the most serious is the inability to make unobtrusive, repeated determinations of BP. Because BP is so variable, one measurement is unreliable. Even taking several measures at one time or on several occasions may not accurately reflect the value of BP over 24 hours. The most important development in recent years in technology to measure BP is the ABPM, which resolves these measurement concerns.

The ABPM device is a small, portable apparatus that allows BP to be measured noninvasively over a 24-hour period. Measurements are made every 10 to 60 minutes. Studies using the ABPM have shown that BP has a diurnal pattern (Pickering, 1992). Blood pressure tends to be lowest during sleep and highest in the afternoon, with a fall in the evening and a rise beginning at about 4 to 6 a.m. Some individuals do not exhibit this fall in BP during the night. These "non-dippers" have a greater degree of left ventricular hypertrophy (Pickering & James, 1993). This finding and other studies (Appel & Stason, 1993; Bottini, Carr, Rhoades, & Prisant, 1992) have led to the supposition that ABPM is a better indicator of target organ damage than the usual episodic BP readings.

Within a research context, ABPM permits comprehensive evaluation of the BP of normotensives and hypertensives, racial groups, males and females, and various age groups and clinical categories (Zachariah, 1992). The ABPM allows BP to be measured during interpersonal interactions, in various settings, and during routine events of normal life. No nursing studies using ABPM were found. This technology has great potential for the examination of BP from a biopsychosocial perspective.

BIOPHYSICAL

Fluid Infusion

Two groups of researchers investigated the efficacy of colloid infusions for treatment of hypovolemia. Howard, Puri, and Paidipaty (1984) found increases in pulmonary artery wedge pressure and mean arterial pressure (MAP) with administration of colloid fluids. Ley and co-workers (Ley, Miller, Shov, & Preisig, 1990) examined hemodynamic stability in cardiac surgery patients. Subjects who received colloid therapy had higher SBP and cardiac outputs postoperatively, as well as shorter ICU lengths of stay. Although the results of these studies persistently favor the use of colloid therapy, it should be noted that the colloid/crystalloid controversy still exists in the critical care community, and continued research is needed.

Presuctioning Oxygenation

Two groups of researchers investigated presuctioning oxygenation and its impact on BP in coronary artery bypass graft (CABG) patients. One group found no significant differences in MAP between the use of a manual resuscitation bag and a ventilator to deliver presuctioning oxygenation (Preusser et al., 1988). These investigators found that the larger the preoxygenation volume (12 vs. 14 cc/kg), the higher the MAP, regardless of method. Other researchers found no significant differences in MAP in those receiving 14 cc/kg as opposed to 12 cc/kg, 16 cc/kg, or 18cc/kg (Stone, Vorst, Lanham, & Zahn, 1989). There was a statistically significant increase of 15 mm Hg in MAP over the three consecutive lung hyperinflation suctioning sequences. These studies demonstrate the value of replication of research to clarify findings.

Patient Position

There have been five studies of the effect of patient position on BP. Several studies of cardiac patients found no significant differences in BP based on lying and chair position. Quaglietti, Stotts, and Lovejoy (1988) studied the effect of sequential positioning at the supine, 70° semi-Fowler, dangle, and chair positions. They found no significant differences in position. No significant differences in MAP were found between the supine and semi-Fowler positions by researchers Kirchhoff, Rebenson-Piano, and Patel (1984). They also found no significant differences in readings when the right atrium or the catheter site was used as a reference point for arterial BP readings. Clochesy (1986) also found no significant differences in SBP and DBP readings in normal patients lying flat, at 45° left and right, and at 35° left and right.

Two researchers examined the differences in BP when lying versus standing. There were no significant differences in the orthostatic SBP response in healthy men and women (Moore & Newton, 1986). Twenty-eight percent of 74 elderly patients attending adult day care showed more evidence of orthostatic hypotension when BP was taken lying than when standing (Walczak, 1991). None of the subjects complained of feeling light-headed or dizzy.

Although the bulk of this literature seems to suggest that changes in position from lying to sitting do not affect BP, the need still exists to study the effect of position on BP in other patient populations. It should also be noted that the researchers who found significant differences based on position were examining the differences between sitting and standing, and only one investigator used only elderly people as subjects. In the other four studies, researchers either did not use elderly subjects (Clochesy, 1986; Moore & Newton, 1986) or combined results from subjects whose ages ranged from 34 to 83 years (Quaglietti et al., 1988) and from 33 to 93 years (Kirchhoff et al., 1984). It is possible that age might have been a confounding variable in these studies.

Medication Administration

Although research related to the choice and dosage of medications is usually performed by other health professionals, three studies were found that included the investigation of the medication administration regimens by nurses. Kremer and Bachenberg (1992) compared BP, heart rate (HR), and sodium nitroprusside (SNP) consumption in post-CABG patients who received either morphine sulfate and midazolam as needed or a continuous infusion of sufentanil and midazolam. They found no significant differences in BP, HR, or SNP consumption between the two groups. Studies that investigate the efficacy of various drug combinations on the reduction of pain and indirectly on BP are an area of direct clinical relevance to nurses. However, these studies should be designed so that each alteration in treatment is evaluated independently. Interactions with other experimental and intervening factors should be examined. For example, the benefits of "standing" as opposed to "as needed" medications would be evaluated independently of the efficacy of one drug over another.

Conant (1988) examined differences in SBP and DBP as a result of nitroglycerin application at four different sites. No significant differences in DBP and plasma nitroglycerin levels were found between sites. Average SBP was lower for the upper arm and anterior chest sites than for the thigh and ankle positions after 75 and 90 minutes. The use of a patient as his or her own research control is an appropriate and practical design for nursing research, as it is usually impossible to design truly experimental studies. However, it is also important to analyze such studies statistically as repeated measures of the same person. Otherwise, the analysis does not fit the design.

Schneider (1987) found no significant differences in SBP, DBP, rate pressure product (RPP), and arrhythmias between those post–myocardial infarction (MI) patients who took a single dose of caffeine compared to those who did not take caffeine.

These studies demonstrated that specific medication therapies, dosage schedules, and application sites can be tested and clarified and remain an important area for future investigation.

Valsalva Maneuver

Metzger and Therrien (1990) and their colleagues have extensively researched the effects of the Valsalva maneuver on BP in various conditions and subjects. There are two phases involved in the Valsalva maneuver, the strain phase and the overshoot phase. Decreases in SBP during straining increases with age in both men and women, but the relationship is significant only with men (Storm, Metzger, & Therrien, 1989). During the straining phase, younger trained individuals had significantly greater decreases in SBP than did older trained subjects (Folta, Metzger, & Therrien, 1989). When these researchers examined the effect of position, with age controlled, the greatest effect of strain on BP was seen when subjects were positioned at 30° and 70°, as opposed to lying flat and or on their right or left sides (Metzger & Therrien, 1990). Increases in SBP during strain were greater for Caucasians than for African Americans and Asians (Lu, Metzger, & Therrien, 1990).

In the overshoot phase there were no significant differences related to age in men and women, but women had significantly greater overshoot of SBP compared to men (Storm, Metzger, & Therrien, 1989). In comparing African Americans, Caucasians, and Asians, Asians had the greatest overshoot (Lu, Metzger, & Therrien, 1990).

This group of researchers has systematically examined the relationship of three important variables, gender, age, and race, on BP during the Valsalva maneuver. Often patients will perform a Valsalva maneuver when changing positions in bed, using a bedpan or commode, or during clinical procedures. Knowledge of the cardiovascular consequences of the Valsalva maneuver allow the nurse to account for its effect and alter nursing routines if necessary.

Movement and Exercise

Six groups of authors described the effects of various activities and exercises on cardiac patients. BP responses to basin baths, tub baths, and showers were compared in a study by Winslow, Lane, and Gaffney (1985). They found that the RPP was similar for all three forms of bathing, but women had higher RPP after tub baths than after showers or basin baths. Stable heart disease patients were studied to compare BP response to occupied versus unoccupied bed making (Harrell et al., 1989). The authors found significantly lower SBP, DBP, and MAP when subjects were in the occupied as opposed to the unoccupied bed positions. The effect of isometric versus nonisometric footboard exercises on normal subjects was compared by Ahrens, Kinney, and Carter (1983). They found no differences in MAP when using these two forms of exercise. These studies highlight the necessity for continued evaluation of effects on BP of what seem "routine" nursing procedures.

Burek and co-workers (Burek, Kirscht, & Topol, 1989) described the effects of early exercise testing on post-MI patients. Subjects with negative treadmill tests had higher SBPs than did those with positive tests, but the difference was not statistically significant. The results of this study indicate that early exercise testing is safe and provides comparable data to standard exercise testing. The effect of graded maximal exercise testing on subjects with established essential hypertension, receiving either a placebo or propranolol, was investigated (Potempa, Folta, Braun, & Szidon, 1992). Results showed that propranolol significantly reduced mean resting and maximal exercise BP. The authors also concluded that clinic resting BP was not a valid predictor of maximal exercise BP. Gillett and Eisenman (1987) found no differences in intensity in controlled and noncontrolled exercise in middle-aged overweight women. The authors found that resting BP did change after the exercise program, but the differences were not significant.

There is a major shift within nursing to change the rationale of clinical practice from a tradition-based model to that of science-based practice. One major task is the evaluation of the effects of nursing interventions on patients. BP is one of the most frequently measured physiological parameters, and therefore BP can easily be used to evaluate the impact of clinical practices on patients. Studies that are carefully designed to answer a specific question about a standard nursing practice will expand to the scientific basis of nursing.

PSYCHOSOCIAL

Pain

Several studies have shown a relationship between decreased pain sensitivity and elevated BP (Ghione, Rosa, Mezzasalma, & Panattoni, 1988; Sheps et al., 1992; Zamir & Shuber, 1980). Bruehl, Carlson, and McCubbin (1992) found that decreased finger pain sensitivity was related to higher resting SBP in 60 normotensive men.

Three articles by the same group of nurse researchers examined BP and pain in the areas of music and imagery (Geden, Lower, Beattie, & Beck, 1989), Lamaze method components (Geden, Beck, Brouder, Glaister, & Pohlmann, 1985), and cognitive-behavioral coping strategies (Geden, Beck, Hague, & Pohlman, 1984) during analogue labor pain in college students. All of the studies used finger pressure pain as the painful stimulus. The use of one experimental method allows for ease in comparison across studies, although one could question the use of finger pressure pain as analogous to labor pain. No significant treatment effects on BP were found. Recent studies determining the relationship of pain sensitivity and BP have suggested one possible explanation for the lack of significance: None of the cited studies accounted for the relationship between resting BP and pain perception. Inclusion of such an analysis might provide a different set of results.

Touch and Massage

Three studies examined the effects of touch and massage on BP. Weiss (1990) examined the effect of touch on adult patients treated for coronary artery disease (CAD) and found that DBP was significantly lower as a result of touch. Hennemen (1989) examined the effect of touch and verbal interaction on patients being weaned from a ventilator. There were no significant effects of touch. MAP was essentially unchanged in both treatment and control groups throughout the experiment. Ferrell-Tory and Glick (1993) examined the effect of massage on inpatients experiencing cancer pain. BP tended to decrease throughout the experiment, and SBP and MAP were significantly lower 10 minutes after the massage on Day 2.

These studies on the effects of touch or massage on BP are recent and inconclusive at this time. They vary widely in the amount and type of touch used, the sample populations, and the surrounding environments of the studies. Careful replication and further research are needed.

Music

The effect of music on BP has been examined in four nursing studies. Two groups of researchers found no significant effect of music on BP, and two had significant results. Zimmerman, Peirson, and Marker (1988) examined the effect of music versus white noise on coronary care unit (CCU) patients. Kaempf and Amodei (1989) reported the effect of listening to classical music with patients who were waiting for surgery. There were no significant differences between groups in these two studies. Steelman (1990) compared the effects of listening to music in patients undergoing surgery with patients who had the usual preoperative surgical care, including verbal distraction to reduce anxiety. There was a significant decrease in BP in the group listening to music. Updike (1990) examined the effect of music on ICU patients and found a significant reduction in SBP and MAP when comparing pre- and post-measurements.

The two studies with significant results (Steelman, 1990; Updike, 1990) allowed the patient to select the type of music. Selection of music reflects individual preferences, and that may have enhanced the effectiveness of the intervention. None of these researchers measured BP before, during, and after the music intervention. This may contribute to the lack of significant effects of music on BP. When studying music interventions, the experimental condition is continuous, and the use multiple measures is mandated during the intervention for complete examination of the response.

Relaxation and Biofeedback

Six studies were found in which investigators examined the effect of relaxation and/or biofeedback training on BP. Pender (1984) taught relaxation in a group setting to patients with hypertension over a period of 6 weeks, followed up at 2 and 4 months later. The relaxation group had significantly lower SBP at 4-month follow-up compared to the control group. The DBP of the relaxation group significantly decreased from baseline but was not significantly different from the control group. Munro, Creamer, Haggerty, and Cooper (1988) examined the effect of relaxation therapy on post-MI patients and compared them to a control group. Relaxation had a significant effect on DBP. Miller and Perry (1990) examined the effectiveness of slow deep breathing on postoperative pain in CABG patients and compared them to a control group. Relaxation was taught the evening before surgery and was performed after surgery. There were significant reductions in SBP and DBP for the experimental group. Warner et al. (1992) examined the effect of relaxation on cardiac catheterization patients. There were no significant differences in the BP of the experimental and the control groups.

The effect of thermal biofeedback and relaxation on the BP of hypertensives was compared to the effect of relaxation only. There was a significant reduction in SBP and DBP in the biofeedback/relaxation group, compared to the relaxation-only group (Hahn et al., 1993). A group of investigators (Nakagawa-Kogan, Garber, Jarrett, Egan, & Hendershot, 1988) examined the characteristics that predict success in a self-regulating BP reduction program for borderline hypertension. They found that lower initial Symptom Check List—90 (SCL-90) scores, lower initial SBP, and higher HR during a mental task could distinguish between those who could and those who could not lower their DBP using a biofeedback/self-management training program.

Nontraditional interventions for management of BP is an innovative and exciting area of nursing research. The studies cited support the extensive literature on the BP-lowering effect of relaxation (Niaura & Goldstein, 1992) and confirm that it is an easily taught technique that can have both long- and short-term effectiveness. Biofeedback research is needed in different populations to determine which patients can benefit from these approaches, which would allow for enhanced effectiveness of the intervention.

Symptom Reporting

Two studies examined the effect of knowledge of BP levels on moods and symptoms. Baumann and Leventhal (1985) compared individuals with DBP above 95 with those who were normotensive and found little relationship between individuals' ability to predict their BP and the subjects' symptoms, moods, and SBP. In the second study, investigators reported three experiments, two of which measured BP (Baumann, Cameron, Zimmerman, & Leventhal, 1989). In the first experiment, undergraduates were given information regarding their BP. The "normal BP biofeedback" group was told their BPs were in the normal range, and the "high BP biofeedback" group was falsely told their BPs were elevated. The effect of this information on symptom reporting was examined. The "high BP biofeedback" group was found to be somewhat more likely to report symptoms of high BP. The second experiment expanded on the first and added the factors of high and low stress levels and beliefs about BP lability. Interactions between stress and beliefs in lability were reported in the "high BP biofeedback" group.

This line of inquiry seeks to determine the relationship between subjective symptom reporting and physical findings. The use of normotensive subjects to test this relationship limits the generalizability of the findings. More research with hypertensive patients and normotensive subjects should be conducted.

Health Belief Model

Three studies were found that examine the relationship of BP to health beliefs. Kerr (1986) examined the relationship between health locus of control and DBP and found that the three-dimensional model of health locus of control (internal, powerful other, and chance) contributed to the prediction of health behavior. The three-dimensional health locus of control orientation accounted for approximately 9% of the variance in DBP. Murdaugh and Verran (1987) tested and expanded the Preventative Behavior Model, an expansion of the Health Belief Model, using SBP and DBP as the outcome variables. Their final empirical model, which included perceived barriers, benefits, health value orientation, and certain health care activities, explained 66% of the variance in SBP and 47% of the variance in DBP. In another study, patients with controlled hypertension were compared to those with uncontrolled hypertension with regard to health beliefs (DeVon & Powers, 1984). No significant differences were found between the groups on compliance potential; however, the patients with uncontrolled hypertension were significantly less adjusted to the illness as measured by higher scores on the Psychosocial Adjustment to Illness Scale.

These studies begin a line of investigation that examines BP from a biopsychosocial perspective and contributes to validation and testing of a middle range theory. The examination of BP as a psychophysiological index is extremely complex and demands more research to elucidate the relationship between the variables involved.

Communication

Several groups of nurse researchers have investigated the effect of communication on BP. Hellman and Grimm (1984) studied hypertensive outpatients who were not taking medication. They found that talking significantly increased DBP, compared to not talking. Liehr (1992) compared BP recorded while the patient listened to a story with BP of a talking patient. Talking resulted in significant increases in BP; listening also significantly increased BP.

Thomas, Lynch, Friedmann, and their colleagues published seven papers between 1983 and 1993 examining the effect of verbal interaction on BP in adults, using a basic protocol called "Quiet-Talk-Quiet." This procedure consisted of measurement of BP with an ABPM once per minute during consecutive minutes of silent resting (quiet), reading or speaking aloud (talk), and silent resting (quiet). In all the studies, BP increased significantly during talking.

Thomas et al. (1984) studied nurses' BP levels before, during, and after shift report and while speaking in front of a small group. Speaking in front of a group caused significantly higher BP than speaking in front of an individual.

Wimbush, Thomas, Friedmann, Sappington, and Lynch (1986) compared the BPs of patients in the cardiac catheterization laboratory (cath lab) and in the patients' rooms after the procedure. Although the patients were sedated, BP was significantly higher in the cath lab during the quiet-talk-quiet procedure than in the patient's room. Freed, Thomas, Lynch, Stein, and Friedmann (1989) again examined the effect of talking on patients with cardiac disease and found that talking significantly increased SBP and DBP. There were no differences in BP between medicated and nonmedicated patients. Thomas and Friedmann (1990) examined Type A behavior and cardiovascular responses to verbalization in cardiac patients but found no relationship between the two factors. Thomas et al. (1992) studied the BP and HR responses of cardiac patients during talking and during an exercise stress test (EST). Systolic BP, DBP, and HR increased significantly during talking. Diastolic BP increased significantly more during talking than during EST stages 1 and 2. HR and SBP increased more during EST than during talking.

Two studies examined the effects of unique types of communication that contained significant nonspoken elements. Malinow, Lynch, Foreman, Friedmann, and Thomas (1986) examined the effect of signing as a type of communication in deaf individuals. They found significant increases in BP during signing, compared to quiet resting periods. Jones and Thomas (1989) described the effect of first-time fathers' interaction with their babies on the BP of the fathers. All measures were significantly higher during interactions with the babies. Frequency of the father's verbal behavior was negatively correlated with SBP, and frequency of infant crying was positively related to the father's DBP. This area of investigation needs to be extended to include more routine nonspoken communication. Patients who are on respirators and must write all of their communications could be examined.

The effect of CCU family visits on patient BP was investigated in two studies (Simpson & Shaver, 1990, 1991). They found no significant differences in MAP, SBP, and DBP between family visits and an interview with the nurse researcher (Simpson & Shaver, 1990). When comparing hypertensive patients to normotensive ones, they found that the hypertensive patients had greater cardiovascular reactivity, though there were no significant differences in BP during family visits and nurse interviews (Simpson & Shaver, 1991).

The BP response to clinical and conversational communication is an area that deserves study. There are many confounding factors that might account for the lack of significant differences based on type of visit, for example, the emotional content of the communication during the visit, the relationship between the patient and the visitor, and the relationship between the patient and the nurse. However, these confounding factors are hard to quantify and control in a research environment. One factor, the amount of time subjects spent talking versus remaining silent, is easily measured.

Companion Animals

Two studies were found on the effects on BP of interacting with a dog. Baun, Bergstrom, Langsten, and Thoma (1984) compared the effect of quiet reading, petting a strange dog, and petting one's own dog on BP, HR, and respiratory rate. Systolic BP and DBP were lowest while petting a companion dog. Gaydos and Farnham (1988) replicated the Baun et al. (1984) study and found no significant differences among the three conditions. The differences between these two studies is minimal, and it is difficult to determine the lack of replication in findings. The effect of being with one's own dog and relaxing with it is difficult to reproduce in an experimental setting. ABPM may be the best method for examining this interaction in the home as it naturally occurs.

CONCLUSION AND FUTURE RESEARCH

Characteristics of the individual, including age, gender, race, health status, SES, occupation, and education, all affect BP. Nursing research has consistently included age, gender, and health status as variables influencing BP. The effects of race and social status have not been examined by nurse researchers although the influence of these variables has been well substantiated by work from other disciplines. The direction of nursing research in BP should be the development of multidimensional models to test the factors within the individual and in the individual's environment, as well as social, economic, and occupational factors that influence an individual's or a group's BP.

The use of auscultatory BP measurements limits the researcher to evaluating BP only as a static cardiovascular variable. Automatic and ambulatory measurement techniques allow exploration into the interpersonal and social aspects of BP and allow repeated measurement of BP under many different conditions. Rather than including multiple measures of BP within each condition, researchers have tended to average BP measures or to make only one measurement for each condition. Use of multiple measures of BP within a condition and the appropriate statistical analysis (such as repeated-measures analysis of variance) capture the dynamic nature of BP. Such analyses statistically account for variances within an individual as well as between individuals, conditions, and groups (Thomas et al., 1993).

Gortner (1990) asserted that nurses should study the physiological aspects of humans in relationship to their health experience and identify the impact of biological, behavioral, social, and cultural conditions. BP research demands this approach if it is to be understood from more than a unidimensional viewpoint. Nursing is uniquely positioned to lead this research on BP from a biopsychosocial perspective.

REFERENCES

Ahrens, W. D., Kinney, M. R., & Carter, R. (1983). The effect of antistasis footboard exercises on selected measures of exertion. *Heart and Lung, 12*, 366–371.

American Heart Association. (1992). *1993 heart and stroke facts statistics*. Dallas, TX: Author.

Appel, L. J., & Stason, W. B. (1993). Ambulatory blood pressure monitoring and blood pressure self-measurement in the diagnosis and management of hypertension. *Annals of Internal Medicine, 118*, 867–882.

Baumann, L. J., Cameron, L. D., Zimmerman, R. S., & Leventhal, H. (1989). Illness representations and matching labels with symptoms. *Health Psychology, 8*, 449–469.

Baumann, L. J., & Leventhal, H. (1985). "I can tell when my blood pressure is up, can't I?" *Health Psychology, 4*, 203–218.

Baun, M. M., Bergstrom, N., Langston, N., & Thoma, L. (1984) . Physiological effects of human/companion animal bonding. *Nursing Research, 33*, 126–129.

Biddle, C. J., & Te, R. (1986). Arm blood pressure gradients in young adults: Impact of induced hypotension. *Heart and Lung, 15*, 588–592.

Bottini, P. B., Carr, A. A., Rhoades, R. B., & Prisant, L. M. (1992). Variability of indirect methods used to determine blood pressure. *Archives of Internal Medicine, 152*, 139–144.

Bruehl, S., Carlson, C. R., & McCubbin, J. A. (1992) . The relationship between pain sensitivity and blood pressure in normotensives. *Pain, 48*, 463–467.

Burek, K. A., Kirscht, J., & Topol, E. J. (1989). Exercise capacity in patients 3 days after acute, uncomplicated myocardial infarction. *Heart and Lung, 18*, 575–580.

Byra-Cook, C. J., Dracup, K. A., & Lazik, A. J. (1990). Direct and indirect blood pressure in critical care patients. *Nursing Research, 39*, 285–288.

Calhoun, D. A. (1992). Hypertension in Blacks: Socioeconomic stress and sympathetic nervous system activity. *American Journal of Medical Sciences, 304*, 306–311.

Chyun, D. A. (1985). A comparison of intra-arterial and auscultatory blood pressure readings. *Heart and Lung, 14*, 223–227.

Clochesy, J. M. (1986). Systemic blood pressure in various lateral recumbent positions: A pilot study. *Heart and Lung, 15*, 593–594.

Conant, C. C. (1988). Plasma nitroglycerin levels, blood pressure and apical heart rate variations to site of application of nitroglycerin ointment. *Nurse Practitioner, 13*(10), 56, 58, 63–64.

DeVon, H. A., & Powers, M. J. (1984). Health beliefs, adjustment to illness, and control of hypertension. *Research in Nursing and Health, 7*, 10–16.

Dressler, W. W. (1990). Education lifestyle and arterial blood pressure. *Journal of Psychosomatic Research, 34*, 515–523.

Ferrell-Torry, A. T., & Glick, O. J. (1993). The use of therapeutic massage as a nursing intervention to modify anxiety and the perception of cancer pain. *Cancer Nursing, 16*, 93–101.

Folta, A., Metzger, B. L., & Therrien, B. (1989). Preexisting physical activity level and cardiovascular responses across the Valsalva maneuver. *Nursing Research, 38*, 139–143.

Freed, C. D., Thomas, S. A., Lynch, J. J., Stein, R., & Friedmann, E. (1989). Blood pressure, heart rate, and heart rhythm changes in patients with heart disease during talking. *Heart and Lung, 18*, 17–22.

Fumo, M. T., Teeger, S., Land, R. M., Bednarz, J., Sareli, P., & Murphy, M. B. (1992). Diurnal blood pressure variation and cardiac mass in American Blacks and Whites and South African blacks. *American Journal of Hypertension, 5*, 111– 116.

Gaydos, L. S., & Farnham, R. (1988). Human-animal relationships within the context of Rogers' principle of integrality. *Advances in Nursing Science, 2*(4), 72–80.

Geddis, M. E., Hoff, H. E., & Badger, S. (1967). Introduction to the auscultatory method of measuring blood pressure including a translation of Korotkoff's original paper. *Cardiovascular Research Bulletin, 5*, 57–74.

Geden, E., Beck, N., Brouder, G., Glaister J., & Pohlman, S. (1985). Self-report and psychophysiological effects of Lamaze preparation: An analogue of labor pain. *Research in Nursing and Health, 8*, 155–165.

Geden, E., Beck, N., Hauge, G., & Pohlman, S. (1984). Self-report and psychophysiological effects of five pain-coping strategies. *Nursing Research, 33*, 260–265.

Geden, E. A., Lower, M., Beattie, S., & Beck, N. (1989). Effects of music and imagery on physiologic and self-report of analogue labor pain. *Nursing Research, 38*, 37–41.

Ghione, S., Rosa, C., Mezzasalma, L., & Panattoni, E. (1988). Arterial hypertension is associated with hypalgesia in humans. *Hypertension, 12*, 491–497.

Gillett, P. A., & Eisenman, P. A. (1987). The effect of intensity controlled aerobic dance exercise on aerobic capacity of middle-aged, overweight women. *Research in Nursing and Health, 10*, 383–390.

Gortner, S. R. (1990). Nursing values and science: Toward a science philosophy. *Image: Journal of Nursing Scholarship, 22*, 101–105.

Hahn, Y. B., Ro, Y. J., Song, H. H., Kim, N. C., Kim, H. S., & Yoo, Y. S. (1993). The effect of thermal biofeedback and progressive muscle training in reducing blood pressure of patients with essential hypertension. *Image: Journal of Nursing Scholarship, 25*, 204–207.

Harrell, J. S., Futrell, A. G., Adams, L. F., Forst, S., Sherwood, A., & Hutcheson, J. S. (1989). Cardiac output and associated cardiovascular responses to bed making. *Critical Care Nursing Quarterly, 12*, 19–33.

Hellmann, R., & Grimm, S. A. (1984). The influence of talking on diastolic blood pressure readings. *Research in Nursing and Health, 7*, 253–256.

Henneman, E. A. (1989). Effect of nursing contact on the stress response of patients being weaned from mechanical ventilation. *Heart and Lung, 18*, 483–489.

Howard, M., Puri, V. K., & Paidipaty, B. B. (1984). The effects of fluid resuscitation in the critically ill patient. *Heart and Lung, 13*, 649–654.

Jones, L. C., & Thomas, S. A. (1989). New fathers' blood pressure and heart rate: Relationships to interaction with their newborn infants. *Nursing Research, 38*, 237–241.

Kaempf, G., & Amodei, M. E. (1989). The effect of music on anxiety. *Association of Operating Room Nurses Journal, 50*, 112–118.

Kerr, J. A. C. (1986). Multidimensional health locus of control, adherence, and lowered diastolic blood pressure. *Heart and Lung, 15*, 87–93.

Kirchhoff, K. T., Rebenson-Piano, M., & Patel, M. K. (1984). Mean arterial pressure readings: Variations with positions and transducer level. *Nursing Research, 33*, 343–345.

Klag, M. J., Whelton, P. K., Coresh, J., Grim, C. E., & Kuller, L. H. (1991). The association of skin color with blood pressure in U.S. Blacks with low socioeconomic status. *Journal of the American Medical Association, 265*, 599–602.

Kremer, M. J., & Bachenberg, K. L. (1992). Sedation by infusion: A clinical trial in cardiac surgery patients. *Journal of the American Association of Nurse Anesthetists, 60,* 354–355.

Ley, S. J., Miller, K., Shov, P., & Preisig, P. (1990). Crystalloid versus colloid fluid therapy after cardiac surgery. *Heart and Lung, 19,* 31–40.

Liehr, P. (1992). Uncovering a hidden language: The effects of listening and talking on blood pressure and heart rate. *Archives of Psychiatric Nursing, 6,* 306–311.

Light, K. C., Obrist, P. A., Sherwood, A., James, S. A., & Strogatz, D. Z. (1987). Effects of race and marginally elevated blood pressure on responses to stress. *Hypertension, 10,* 555–563.

Long, J., Lynch, J. J., Machiran, N. M., Thomas, S. A., & Malinow, K. (1982). The effect of status on blood pressure during verbal communication. *Journal of Behavioral Medicine, 5,* 165–172.

Lu, Z., Metzger, B. L., & Therrien, B. (1990). Ethnic differences in physiological responses associated with the Valsalva maneuver. *Research in Nursing and Health, 13,* 9–15.

Malinow, K. L., Lynch, J. J., Foreman, P. J., Friedmann, E., & Thomas, S. A. (1986). Blood pressure increases while signing in a deaf population. *Psychosomatic Medicine, 48,* 95–101.

Mauro, A. M. P. (1988). Effects of bell versus diaphragm on indirect blood pressure measurement. *Heart and Lung, 17,* 489–494.

Metzger, B. L., & Therrien, B. (1990). Effect of position on cardiovascular response during the Valsalva maneuver. *Nursing Research, 39,* 198–202.

Miller, K. M., & Perry, P. P. (1990). Relaxation technique and postoperative pain in patients undergoing cardiac surgery. *Heart and Lung, 19,* 136–146.

Moore, K. I., & Newton, K. (1986). Orthostatic heart rates and blood pressures in healthy young women and men. *Heart and Lung, 15,* 611–617.

Munro, B. H., Creamer, A. M., Haggerty, M. R., & Cooper, F. S. (1988). Effect of relaxation therapy on post-myocardial infarction patients' rehabilitation. *Nursing Research, 37,* 231–235.

Murdaugh, C. L., & Verran, J. A. (1987). Theoretical modeling to predict physiological indicant of cardiac preventive behaviors. *Nursing Research, 36,* 284–291.

Nakagawa-Kogan, H., Garber, A., Jerrett, M., Egan, K. J., & Hendershot, S. (1988). Self-management of hypertension: Predictors of success in diastolic blood pressure reduction. *Research in Nursing and Health, 11,* 105–115.

Niaura, R., & Goldstein, M. G. (1992). Psychological factors affecting physical conditions: Part 2. Coronary artery disease and sudden death and hypertension. *Psychosomatics, 33,* 146–155.

Pender, N. J. (1984). Physiologic responses of clients with essential hypertension to progressive muscle relaxation training. *Research in Nursing and Health, 7,* 197–203.

Pickering, T. (1992). Ambulatory blood pressure monitoring: An historical perspective. *Clinical Cardiology, 15*(Suppl. 1), 113–115.

Pickering, T. G., & James, G. D. (1989). Some implications of the differences between home, clinic, and ambulatory blood pressure in normotensive and hypertensive patients. *American Journal of Hypertension, 7*(Suppl. 7), S65–S72.

Pickering, T. G., James, G. D. (1993). Determinants and consequences of the diurnal rhythm of blood pressure. *American Journal of Hypertension, 6,* S166–S169.

Potempa, K. M., Folta, A., Braun, L. T., & Szidon, J. P. (1992). The relationship of resting and exercise blood pressure in subjects with essential hypertension before and after drug treatment with propranolol. *Heart and Lung, 21,* 509–514.

Preusser, B. A., Stone, K. S., Bonyon, D. S., Winningham, M. L., Groch, K. F., & Karl, J. E. (1988). Effects of two methods of preoxygenation on mean arterial pressure, cardiac output, peak airway pressure, and postsuctioning hypoxemia. *Heart and Lung, 17,* 290–298.

Quaglietti, S. E., Stotts, N. A., & Lovejoy, N. C. (1988). The effect of selected positions on rate pressure product of the post myocardial infarction patient. *Journal of Cardiovascular Nursing, 2*(4), 77–85.

Rebenson-Piano, M., Holm, K., Foreman, M. D., & Kirchhoff, K. T. (1989). An evaluation of two indirect methods of blood pressure measurement in ill patients. *Nursing Research, 38,* 42–45.

Rebenson-Piano, M., Holm, K., & Powers, M. (1987). An examination of the differences that occur between direct and indirect blood pressure measurement. *Heart and Lung, 16,* 285–294.

Rieser, M. F., Reeves, R. B., & Armington, J. (1958). Effect of variations in laboratory procedure and experimenter upon the ballistocardiograph, blood pressure and heart rate in healthy young men. *Psychosomatic Medicine, 17,* 185–189.

Saunders, E. (1991). Hypertension in blacks. *Primary Care, 18,* 607–621.

Schneider, J. R. (1987). Effects of caffeine ingestion on blood pressure, myocardial oxygen consumption, and cardiac rhythm in acute myocardial infarction patients. *Heart and Lung, 16,* 167–174.

Sheps, D. S., Bragdon, E. E., Gray, T. F., Ballenger, M., Usedom, J. E., & Maixner W. (1992). Relationship between systemic hypertension and pain perception. *American Journal of Cardiology, 70*(16 Suppl.), 3F–5F.

Simpson, T., & Shaver, J. (1990). Cardiovascular responses to family visits in coronary care unit patients. *Heart and Lung, 19,* 344–351.

Simpson, T., & Shaver, J. (1991). A comparison of hypertensive and nonhypertensive coronary care patients' cardiovascular responses to visitors. *Heart and Lung, 20,* 213–220.

Steelman, V. M. (1990). Intraoperative music therapy. *Association of Operating Room Nurses Journal, 52,* 1026–1034.

Stone, K. S., Vorst, E. C., Lanham, B., & Zahn, S. (1989). Effects of lung hyperinflation on mean arterial pressure and postsuctioning hypoxemia. *Heart and Lung, 18,* 377–385.

Storm, D. S., Metzger, G. L., & Therrien, B. (1989). Effects of age on autonomic cardiovascular responsiveness in healthy men and women. *Nursing Research, 38,* 326–330.

Tachovsky, B. J. (1985). Indirect auscultatory blood pressure measurement at two sites in the arm. *Research in Nursing and Health, 8,* 125–129.

Thomas, S. A., Freed, C. D., Friedmann, E., Stein, R., Lynch, J. J., & Rosch, P. J. (1992). Cardiovascular responses of patients with cardiac disease to talking and exercise stress testing. *Heart and Lung, 21,* 64–73.

Thomas, S. A., & Friedmann, E. (1990). Type A behavior and cardiovascular response during verbalization in cardiac patients. *Nursing Research, 39,* 48–53.

Thomas, S. A., Friedmann, E., Lottes, L. S., Gresty, S., Miller, C., & Lynch, J. J. (1984). Changes in nurses' blood pressure while communicating. *Research in Nursing and Health, 7,* 119–126.

Thomas, S. A., Liehr, P., DeKeyser, F., & Friedmann, E. (1993). Nursing blood pressure research, 1980–1990: A bio-psycho-social perspective. *Image: Journal of Nursing Scholarship*, *25*, 157–164.

Updike, P. (1990). Music therapy results for ICU patients. *Dimensions of Critical Care Nursing*, *9*, 39–45.

Walczak, M. (1991). Prevalence of orthostatic hypotension. *Journal of Gerontological Nursing*, *17*(11), 26–29.

Warner, C. D., Peebles, B. U., Miller, J., Reed, R., Rodriquez, S., & Martin-Lewis, E. (1992). The effectiveness of teaching a relaxation technique to patients undergoing cardiac catheterization. *Journal of Cardiovascular Nursing*, *6*(2), 66–75.

Weiss, S. J. (1990). Effects of differential touch on nervous system arousal of patients recovering from cardiac disease. *Heart and Lung*, *19*, 474–480.

Willius, F. A., & Keys, T. E. (1941). *Classics of cardiology*, New York: Dover.

Wimbush, F. B., Thomas, S. A., Friedmann, E., Sappington, E., & Lynch, J. J. (1986). Cardiovascular responses to communication during catheterization. *Dimensions of Critical Care Nursing*, *5*, 244–250.

Winslow, E. H., Lane, L. D., & Gaffney, F. A. (1985). Oxygen uptake and cardiovascular responses in control adults and acute myocardial infarction patients during bathing. *Nursing Research*, *34*, 164–169.

Zachariah, P. (1992). The role of ambulatory blood pressure monitoring in research. *Clinical Cardiology*, *15*(Suppl. 1), 116–119.

Zamir, N., & Shuber, E. (1980). Altered pain perception in hypertensive humans. *Brain Research*, *201*, 471–474.

Zimmerman, L. M., Pierson, M. A., & Marker, J. (1988). Effects of music on patient anxiety in coronary care units. *Heart and Lung*, *17*, 560–566.

Chapter 2

Psychoneuroimmunological Studies in HIV Disease

NANCY L. MCCAIN
SCHOOL OF NURSING
VIRGINIA COMMONWEALTH UNIVERSITY

JANICE M. ZELLER
RUSH UNIVERSITY COLLEGE OF NURSING

CONTENTS

A number of psychobiological stimuli under the general rubric of stress have been reported to influence immune function (Herzberg, Murtaugh, & Beitz, 1994; Khansari, Murgo, & Faith, 1990; O'Leary, 1990; Weisse, 1992). Much of this research has recently been conducted using the framework of psychoneuroimmunology (PNI), which is concerned with bidirectional communication between the neuroendocrine and immune systems (Rabin, Cohen, Ganguli, Lysle, & Cunnick, 1989). The majority of PNI studies to date have been focused either on relationships between stress and illness, implying an immunological linkage (Cohen & Williamson, 1991), or between stress and immunity, with the suggestion of health implications (Herbert & Cohen, 1993b).

Few researchers have attempted simultaneous investigations of relationships among these three concepts (e.g., Cohen, Tyrrell, & Smith, 1991; Glaser et al., 1987; Levy, Herberman, Maluish, Schlien, & Lippman, 1985). Most recently, PNI research has been focused on the influence of biobehavioral strategies on immunological outcomes in healthy subjects as well as clinical populations (Kiecolt-Glaser & Glaser, 1992; Schulz & Schulz, 1992). Although most PNI studies have characterized the influence of psychological factors on immunity, growing numbers of scientists are examining the modulation of neuroendocrine functioning by immune-derived products (Blalock, 1992; Reichlin, 1993). It is anticipated that a more thorough understanding of this bidirectional communication network will shed light on the mechanisms potentially underlying certain neuroendocrine as well as immunological disturbances. (For comprehensive reviews on PNI, please see Ader, Felton, & Cohen, 1991; Kiecolt-Glaser & Glaser, 1994; Newberry, Jaikins-Madden, & Gerstenberger, 1991; Plotnikoff, Murgo, Faith, & Wybran, 1991).

PNI research with human subjects has involved numerous populations, including individuals grieving the death of a loved one (Calabrese, Kling, & Gold, 1987), persons caring for a spouse with dementia (Kiecolt-Glaser, Dura, Speicher, Trask, & Glaser, 1991), students undergoing examination stress (Glaser et al., 1991), cancer patients, (Levy et al., 1985), and many others (Kiecolt-Glaser et al., 1987; Palmblad, Petrini, Wasserman, & Åkerstedt, 1979; Schleifer, Keller, Bond, Cohen, & Stein, 1989). Although persons infected with the human immunodeficiency virus (HIV) have only recently become participants in PNI research, several reviews have been written on this subject (e.g., Antoni et al., 1990; Gorman & Kertzner, 1990; Kemeny, 1994a, 1994b; Solomon, Kemeny, & Temoshok, 1991). HIV disease is an ideal illness to study from a PNI perspective because it is an infectious disease that theoretically can be inactivated by immunological mechanisms; it is a disease that results in progressive immunological dysfunction, leading to increased susceptibility to opportunistic infections and malignancies; and it involves a clinical picture that may include psychological and neuroendocrinological disturbances (Solomon, 1987; Solomon & Temoshok, 1987). Persons infected with HIV experience a clinical course that is highly variable, although it is estimated that most persons develop the acquired immune deficiency syndrome (AIDS) within 10 to 15 years postinfection (Weiss, 1993). A number of factors have been proposed to account for this variable disease course, including host genetic features, virulence of the viral strain, nutritional status, and psychosocial factors (Guenter et al., 1993; Levy, 1994; Livingston, 1988; Taylor, 1994).

This review is focused on PNI studies in HIV disease. Relevant research was defined as reports of studies (including published abstracts with sufficient information to interpret study findings) of persons with HIV disease, published in English from 1987 through 1994 and aimed at psychosocial phenomena and their associations with the immune system and/or related health outcomes. Publications that were purely descriptive or only psychological in nature were not included in the review. Computerized search strategies included citations from MEDLINE, AIDSLINE, Cumulative Index to Nursing and Allied Health Literature (CINAHL), and PsycINFO, retrieved with combinations of the keywords PNI, HIV/AIDS, psychological stress, and/or psychophysiology (with immunology). Articles also were identified from review references and through research ancestry. Finally, manuscripts known to be in press were obtained, if possible, from the authors. Following a brief review of the immune system and the pathogenesis of HIV infection in the context of PNI, 36 studies are reviewed.

HIV DISEASE AND PSYCHONEUROIMMUNOLOGY

The function of the immune system is to recognize infectious organisms and abnormal host cells and eliminate them from the body. These activities are carried out by nonspecific effector cells, including phagocytic cells (e.g., granulocytes, monocytes, and macrophages) and natural killer (NK) cells, which destroy tumors and virally infected target cells. In addition, specific mechanisms such as cell-mediated or humoral immune reactions may be called into play. T lymphocytes participate in cell-mediated immune reactions against tumor cells and, in conjunction with macrophages, generate delayed-type hypersensitivity reactions to infectious parasites. B lymphocytes generate antibody in response to viral and bacterial infections. All immune reactions are under the regulation of two categories of T lymphocytes: T helper (CD4+) cells and T suppressor (CD8+) cells. The relative numbers and functional activities of these lymphocyte populations influence the strength and persistence of an immune response. (For comprehensive discussions of the immune system, see Abbas, Lichtman, & Pober, 1994; Kuby, 1994; Roitt, Brostoff, & Male, 1993).

The primary target for HIV infection is the CD4+ T helper/inducer lymphocyte (Stein, Korvick, & Vermund, 1992), a cell that plays a key role in orchestrating both cell-mediated and humoral immune mechanisms. Once CD4+ T lymphocytes are infected with HIV, the virus may remain dormant or undergo replication, resulting in dysfunction and ultimate death of the CD4+ target cell (Miedema, Tersmette, & van Lier, 1990). It has been proposed that HIV replication within CD4+ T lymphocytes requires an actively proliferating cell (Stevenson, Stanwick, Dempsey, & Lamonica, 1990; Zack et al., 1990). Recent data from two independent laboratories has revealed that HIV disease represents a dynamic process whereby CD4+ T lymphocytes are continuously infected, destroyed, and newly generated (Ho et al., 1995; Wei et al., 1995). A decline in CD4+ lymphocyte counts occurs when the proportional rate of cell destruction exceeds cell replication.

Because mononuclear phagocytes like T helper lymphocytes express the CD4 marker on their surface, they also are infected by HIV (Gartner et al., 1986; Koenig et al., 1986; Nicholson, Cross, Callaway, & McDougal, 1986). Tissue mononuclear phagocytes (macrophages) may be more susceptible than blood monocytes to infection with HIV and further viral propagation (Gendelman & Meltzer, 1989). Unlike CD4+ T lymphocytes, however, mononuclear phagocytes are not destroyed by HIV infection but appear to serve as long-term reservoirs for the virus (Pauza, 1988; Roy & Wainberg, 1988).

A decline in CD4+ T lymphocyte numbers over the course of illness has been considered to be the hallmark of HIV disease progression (Stein et al., 1992). T helper cell function is reduced, as evidenced by decreased ability of lymphocytes to proliferate in response to antigens or mitogens in culture (Clerici et al., 1989) or to undergo a delayed-type hypersensitivity response in vivo (Blatt et al., 1993). Other immunological changes that occur in association with disease progression include alterations in numbers of CD8+ cytotoxic/suppressor T lymphocytes (Cooper, Tindall, Wilson, Imrie, & Penny, 1988; Lang et al., 1989; Watret, Whitelaw, Froebel, & Bird, 1993) and an increase in expression of cellular activation markers (CD38, HLA-DR, and CD69) on CD8+ cells (Hulstaert et al., 1992). Diminished functioning of NK cells, as well as reduced cell numbers (identified by CD16 and/or CD56 surface markers), are seen over the course of HIV disease (Brenner, Dascal, Margolese, & Wainberg, 1989).

In contrast to the reduction in cell-mediated immunity evidenced by reduced T lymphocyte and NK cell activities, there is evidence of B cell hyperreactivity in association with HIV disease (Lane et al., 1983). Additionally, there may be general immune system stimulation, as evidenced by elevated levels of the cellular activation products β_2-microglobulin and neopterin (Fahey et al., 1990; Melmed, Taylor, Bozorgmehri, & Fahey, 1989; Schwartländer, Bek, Skarabis, & Koch for the Multicentre Cohort Study Group, 1993). These seemingly paradoxical findings may be the result of an immunological dysregulation, reflected by changes in cytokine secretion by immune cells. As HIV disease progresses, there appears to be a shift from a predominant type 1 cytokine response (mediated by interleukin [IL]-2, IL-12, and gamma-interferon), which favors cell-mediated immune reactions, to a predominant type 2 response (mediated by IL-4, IL-5, IL-6, and IL-10), which favors humoral immune responses (Clerici & Shearer, 1993; Shearer & Clerici, 1992). With the progression of immunological dysfunction, HIV titer (viral burden) increases (Piatak et al., 1993; Schnittman et al., 1990).

There is some accumulating evidence that the psychological stress associated with being infected with HIV may accelerate the course of illness

(Mulder & Antoni, 1992; Schneiderman et al., 1993; Solomon et al., 1991). Based on both clinical and psychometric evidence, HIV-infected persons may experience a high degree of stress (Folkman, 1993; LaPerriere, Antoni, et al., 1991; Strawn, 1991). It is plausible that elevated levels of cortisol associated with stress may accelerate the course of illness, either by suppressing the function of immune cells that carry out antiviral activities (Migliorati et al., 1994), by encouraging a predominant type 2 as opposed to type 1 cytokine response pattern (Clerici et al., 1994), or by enhancing HIV replication in infected cells through binding to the steroid response element in the HIV viral genome (Kolesnitchenko & Snart, 1992). Stress induces the escape of herpes viruses from latency, as evidenced by elevated serum antiviral antibodies (Glaser et al., 1987), and may have a similar effect on HIV (Glaser & Kiecolt-Glaser, 1987). It is additionally plausible that, by allowing reexpression of previously latent viruses or facilitating host infection with new viruses, stress will result in immune cell stimulation and thus enhanced replication of HIV (Schneiderman et al., 1994). Although there are numerous mechanisms whereby stress hormones may directly influence HIV disease progression, acting at the level of the immune cell or HIV viral genome, it also is possible that behavioral changes associated with stress (e.g., changes in eating patterns, sleep, or drug use) may contribute to disease progression (Kemeny, 1994a). Given these multiple potential mechanisms, the associations among psychosocial factors, neuroendocrine and immune functioning, and health status have become important research foci in HIV disease.

REVIEW OF RESEARCH

A total of 36 studies was identified as relevant to this review of PNI studies in HIV disease; of these, 6 were conducted by nurses. Studies were broadly categorized by major conceptual focus or purpose as stress and coping (10), psychological distress (14), psychological well-being (5), and interventions (7). All statistically significant findings reported in this review were at the $p \le .05$ level.

Stress and Coping

For some time the associations among stress, coping, and illness have been major areas of interest in PNI. More recently, stress and coping effectiveness have been considered as cofactors for progression of HIV disease. In one of the earlier PNI-related studies, Namir, Wolcott, Fawzy, and Alumbaugh (1987) examined patterns of coping among 50 gay men with AIDS. Avoidance coping [using their Dealing with Illness–coping inventory (Namir et al., 1987)] was associated with greater depression and anxiety [on the Profile of Mood States (McNair, Lorr, & Droppleman, 1971)] and lower social support and self-esteem, whereas active-behavioral coping was related to less total mood disturbance and depression and higher social support and self-esteem. Although self-perceived health status was positively related to active-behavioral coping and negatively related to avoidance coping, neither physician ratings of performance capacity nor medical symptoms were correlated with coping patterns. Although this early study was limited to gay men with AIDS, it provided some insight and direction for future intervention studies.

Stress and coping have been major areas of interest in the Center for the Biopsychosocial Study of AIDS at the University of Miami. Blaney et al. (1991) described the framework for this research in a report on a stress-moderator model of psychological distress. The 5-year longitudinal study of gay men with HIV disease included repeated measures of life stressors, coping styles, hardiness, social support, and psychological distress. In the first follow-up report for 68 asymptomatic and 22 symptomatic men, Blaney et al. (1992) reported that negative life events, as indicated by the Life Experiences Survey (Sarason, Johnson, & Siegel, 1978), and active coping, using the Coping Orientations to Problems Experienced scale (Carver, Scheier, & Weintraub, 1989), predicted the number of HIV-related symptoms over a 6-month period, with stress positively associated and coping negatively correlated with symptoms. Goodkin and colleagues (Goodkin, Blaney, et al. 1992, 1993; Goodkin, Fuchs, Feaster, Leeka, & Rishel, 1992) and Blaney et al. (1991, 1992) have continued to report longitudinal findings with this cohort.

In a sample of 62 HIV-seropositive homosexual men (without AIDS), Goodkin, Blaney, et al. (1992) found a positive relationship between NK cell cytotoxicity and an active coping style. Although the relationships did not achieve significance, there were trends toward an inverse association of NK cell cytotoxicity with life stressors and a positive moderating effect of social support on stress levels. It is noteworthy that Goodkin, Blaney, et al. found significant effects only when control variables for alcohol use and nutritional status (which together accounted for 42% of the variance in cytotoxicity) were included in the regression models.

Goodkin's group (Goodkin, Fuchs, et al., 1992) also reported preliminary work using the Life Experience Survey and the Millon Behavioral Health Inventory (Millon, Green, & Meagher, 1982) for coping styles. With a pilot sample of 11 HIV-infected men, significant relationships were found between higher stress and passive coping style as well as lower total lymphocyte counts. In the most recent Goodkin et al. (Goodkin, Blaney, et al., 1993) report, for an expanded sample of 103 asymptomatic and early symptomatic gay men, long-term (up to 3.5 years) CD4$^+$ cell count was negatively related to stress levels and a passive coping style, using the Coping Orientations to Problems Experienced scale.

In contrast to these findings, Kessler et al. (1991) concluded that there was no evidence that serious stressor events play a meaningful part in symptom onset, defined as a 25% decline in CD4$^+$ percentage in 6 months and/or onset of thrush or fever lasting at least 2 weeks. Subjects were gay men recruited for the Coping and Change Study at the Chicago site of the Multicenter AIDS Cohort Study; the sample size for these analyses was not clear. The nature of the stressors assessed also was not clear, described only as the number of AIDS diagnoses and/or deaths in the subject's network and frequency scores on a 24-item checklist of "more general serious stressor events" (p. 734). Of concern in this study as reported is questionable measurement validity. A 25% decline in CD4$^+$ percentage is equivalent to the *annual* decline reported for participants in the Multicenter AIDS Cohort Study in Chicago (MacDonnell, Chmiel, Poggensee, Wu, & Phair, 1990). Further confounding measurement validity, the percentage of decline was analyzed only for those subjects with baseline percentages of 45 or more (i.e., those less likely to progress over the 3.5-year study period). Numbers of participants declining by 25% were essentially equal in HIV-seropositive and HIV-seronegative groups, verifying a lack of discriminant validity.

Evans et al. (1991) provided a preliminary report on 35 HIV-seronegative and 24 asymptomatic HIV-seropositive gay men enrolled in the Coping in Health and Illness Project (CHIP) in North Carolina. In this group, there were negative relationships between stress (as measured by a new interview scale) and NK cell count and percentage in the HIV-infected group. The HIV-positive men also had higher stress levels than those of the seronegative comparison group. Evans, Leserman, Perkins, Murphy, and Folds (1992) later reported findings related to social support as a stress moderator for the cohort of gay men enrolled in CHIP. For the 63 HIV-seropositive subjects, scores for number of supportive relationships on Sarason and colleagues' (1987) social support measure correlated positively with percentage of CD4$^+$ cells and negatively with percentage of CD8$^+$ cells.

Psychological Distress

A large body of research supports a relationship between stress and psychological distress (often indicated by depression), mediated, in part, by the individual's perception of the meaning and importance of potentially stressful events (Gruen, 1993). Although there is a tendency for indicators of psychological distress to be implicitly or explicitly considered as sufficient evidence of stress, the concepts of stress and distress are not interchangeable, with distress generally considered to be a response to stress (Derogatis & Coons, 1993).

Kemeny and colleagues at the University of California, Los Angeles (UCLA), Multicultural AIDS Cohort Study site have been interested in relationships among immune parameters and depression in the context of bereavement, as well as specific patterns of coping with HIV disease. In comparisons of bereaved versus nonbereaved and HIV-seropositive versus HIV-seronegative gay men ($N = 90$), Kemeny et al. (1994) found significant associations with immune parameters only in the nonbereaved group of HIV-infected men. In the latter group, higher depressed mood (on the Profile of Mood States) was related to lower CD4$^+$ cell percentages, higher percentages of CD8$^+$CD38$^+$ T cells, and lower lymphocyte proliferation responses. Contrary to study hypotheses, depression was not significantly related to any immune parameter among the bereaved HIV-infected men. Among the seronegative subjects only, depression was inversely associated with the percentage of NK (CD16$^+$) cells. Potential explanations for the nonsignificant findings in bereaved individuals include psychological adaptation to repeated bereavement and inadequate timing of measurements in relation to personal losses.

The UCLA group also reported a prospective psychobiological study of 74 gay men with AIDS, in which a pattern of coping characterized as realistic acceptance was found to predict median survival time, which was decreased by 9 months in those with high realistic acceptance scores on this factor (Reed, Kemeny, Taylor, Wang, & Visscher, 1994). Realistic acceptance, as measured by the Responses to HIV scale [an adaptation of the Lazarus Ways of Coping Checklist (Folkman & Lazarus, 1980)], was not correlated with psychological distress or dispositional optimism and significantly predicted reduced survival time beyond the influence of self-reported health status or CD4$^+$ cell count. According to the investigators, "Realistic Acceptance appears to represent a fundamentally cognitive phenomenon, and to be a function of negative disease-specific expectancies in the context of AIDS" (p. 305). Although presented as a prospective study, the methods do not fully support that interpretation. For example, CD4$^+$ cell counts were from clinical blood draws ($n = 48$) at the most recent Multicultural AIDS Cohort Study visit within 6 months prior to questionnaire completion. Thus, timing of CD4$^+$ cell counts in relation to questionnaire completion was, presumably, highly variable.

Perry, Fishman, Jacobsberg, and Frances (1992), of Cornell University, reported correlational data with a 1-year follow-up for 221 HIV-seropositive subjects without AIDS in New York City. There were no concurrent nor prospective relationships among CD4$^+$ T lymphocyte levels and the psychosocial variables of depression, anxiety, psychological distress, stressful life events, hardiness, social support, and bereavement. Only an index of hopelessness, derived from specific items of the Brief Symptom Inventory (BSI) (Derogatis & Melisaratos, 1983) and the Beck Depression Inventory (BDI) (Beck, Ward, & Mendelson, 1961), was found to predict the CD4$^+$ cell count at 6 months. Additionally, emotional distress, as indicated by multiple measures, was positively associated with HIV-related physical symptoms.

In a similar correlational study conducted by researchers at the New York State Psychiatric Institute with 124 HIV-seropositive gay men without AIDS, Rabkin et al. (1991) found no concurrent or predictive relationships at 6 months among depression, anxiety, global psychological distress, social support, bereavement, or stressful life events and either HIV-related symptoms or T lymphocyte subsets. The investigators noted that only a small fraction of their sample (17%) could be indexed as depressed, and the mean scores on all measures of psychological distress and stressful life events were low for the sample as a whole, thus restricting the range of scores for the analyses. Significant declines were noted over time, not only for health status but also for several measures of stress levels and psychological distress.

In the second baseline publication for the New York psychiatric group, Gorman et al. (1991) reported that mean levels of 24-hour urinary free cortisol were positively correlated with HIV-related symptoms and medical stage of illness and with depression and anxiety but were not significantly related to CD4$^+$ or CD8$^+$ T lymphocyte levels. However, the overall degree of hypothalamic-pituitary-adrenal axis activation, as evidenced by levels of urinary free cortisol, was minimal for this sample. Thus, cortisol levels might not have been of a sufficient magnitude to measurably affect immune function in this relatively healthy sample. Kertzner et al. (1993) reported that the baseline correlations for urinary cortisol did not remain significant over the next 2 years of follow-up with this cohort. Cortisol levels were not significantly different for HIV-seropositive ($n = 109$) and HIV-seronegative ($n = 75$) men at any time, although there was a strong trend for declining urinary cortisol over time in those with HIV infection. At 3 years into the study, there were no meaningful relationships among the psychological measures and NK (CD56$^+$) cells (Sahs et al., 1994). This cohort of men remained fairly healthy and generally lacked psychopathology.

Among 81 people at various stages of HIV disease, Robertson et al. (1993) examined the relationship between psychological distress and antibody titers to herpes viruses, including cytomegalovirus, Epstein-Barr virus, and herpes simplex virus. Greater psychological distress (as indicated by the POMS and the BSI) was correlated with higher herpes simplex antibody titers, indicating less immunological control of viral replication. It is possible that distress could alter HIV disease progression by causing reactivation of latent herpes simplex virus, which could then potentiate HIV replication. There were no significant relationships among the psychological variables and cytomegalovirus or Epstein-Barr virus titers nor CD4+ cell count. However, high mean levels of cytomegalovirus and Epstein-Barr virus antibodies in this sample might have masked correlations by restricting the range of observations.

Two correlational studies more specifically concerned with depression were published simultaneously in the *Journal of the American Medical Association*: Burack and associates (1993) reported on the San Francisco Men's Health Study, and the Lyketsos group (1993) represented the Multicultural AIDS Cohort Study. Burack et al. (1993) found that among 277 HIV-infected gay men without AIDS who were followed for up to 5 years, those classified as depressed on the affective items of the Center for Epidemiological Studies–Depression scale (CES-D) (Radloff, 1977) had a 34% greater mean annual rate of decline in CD4+ counts (−80 vs. −60 cells/microliter/year). The differential decline in CD4+ levels was not attributable to differences in baseline CD4+ counts, antiretroviral medication use, recreational drug or alcohol use, symptomatology, or the individual's knowledge of his HIV status (because all subjects were unaware of their seropositive status at the time of the depression measurement). To analyze CD4 decline, a linear regression coefficient was calculated from a minimum of three cell counts (and up to 12 data points) for each subject to represent the individual's annual rate of decline.

With a cohort of 1,339 HIV-seropositive gay men who were without AIDS and demographically quite similar to those in the Burack (1993) study, Lyketsos et al. (1993) found no difference between depressed and nondepressed subjects in the rate of CD4+ T lymphocyte decline or other progression indicators for the 5-year follow-up period. However, depressed participants (21.3% with CES-D ≥16) had lower CD4+ counts and more HIV-related symptoms at baseline than did those who were not depressed. The mean decline in CD4+ count for the group was 28–29 cells/microliter over 6 months. CD4 decline was defined by individual regression slopes calculated from a minimum of 5 (and up to 13) cell counts taken every 6 months.

In an editorial concerning these two studies, Perry and Fishman (1993) contended that the findings were probably of no clinical significance, many confounds were not controlled, the reported statistical significance could be due to chance (type I error), and calculation of the CD4 decline using five measures tended to enhance reliability in the Lyketsos et al. (1993) study. Perry and Fishman (1993) concluded that "the development of HIV-related physical symptoms increases the likelihood of depression, but that depressive symptoms do not in themselves increase the progression of HIV disease"

(p. 2610). Given that both groups of investigators measured depressed mood rather than clinical depression and neither group assessed psychological treatment over time, study findings would tend to be biased toward the null hypotheses. Additionally, the smaller sample in the Burack et al. (1993) study resulted in relatively less statistical power, further biasing that study toward a type II error. Although these study findings are controversial, a 10% higher death rate after 5 years among those who were depressed (Burack et al., 1993) argues for the clinical significance of depressed mood. Debate regarding these conflicting studies of depression as a cofactor in HIV disease has continued, with additional editorial comments in Barrett et al. (1994) and Lyketsos, Hoover, and Guccione (1994).

Based on an explicit PNI framework, Nokes and Kendrew (1990) examined the relationship of loneliness [as measured by the Differential Loneliness Scale (Schmidt & Sermat, 1983)] to the frequency of infections over 6 months in 31 men with AIDS. No significant relationship was found, and there was no overall increase in loneliness (although the romantic/sexual loneliness subscale was increased) over the study period. Findings in this study could be attributable to a testing effect, with measures repeated every month for 6 months.

With 156 individuals at various stages of HIV disease, Linn, Monnig, Cain, and Usoh (1993) found that self-reported stage of illness was not significantly related to sense of coherence [using the Perceived Coherence scale (Lewis & Gallison, 1989) instrument], depression, or anxiety. However, increased physical symptomatology was associated with higher depression (on the CES-D) and anxiety [using the Anxiety Scale (Lewis, Firsich, & Parsell, 1979)] and lower sense of coherence. Sense of coherence also was inversely correlated with depression and anxiety. Because study hypotheses were contradictory in some respects, the authors' expectations regarding the nature of these relationships in the context of HIV-disease progression were not clear. Measurement validity issues include self-reported stage of illness and social support measured as the number of confidants (with no measure of satisfaction with or quality of social support).

McCain and Cella (1995) found that among 53 men at various stages of HIV disease, higher levels of negative-impact stress were correlated with lower quality of life; higher psychological distress, as indicated by a brief form of the POMS (Cella et al., 1987) and the Impact of Event Scale (IES) (Horowitz, Wilner, & Alvarez, 1979); more uncertainty (on the Mishel Uncertainty in Illness Scale [Mishel, 1981; 1984]) and more frequent use of an emotion-focused coping pattern. Quality of life was inversely related to psychological distress, uncertainty, and emotion-focused coping. Lower CD4$^+$ cell counts were associated only with increased positive-impact stress, a potentially spurious relationship in this study. Stress and coping were measured by the Dealing with Illness Scale (McCain & Gramling, 1992) (a population-specific form of the LES), and quality of life was assessed by the Functional Assessment of HIV Infection scale (Cella, 1992).

In a study of 30 men with AIDS by van Servellen, Padilla, Brecht, and Knoll (1993), depression (defined by the CES-D) was directly related to stress levels (on the LES) and numbers of clinical health problems and inversely related to the stress-resistance resources of social support, using Sarason's scale (Sarason, Sarason, Potter, & Antoni, 1985) and intrapersonal hope on the Stoner Hope Scale (Stoner, 1982). There were no significant correlations between CD4+ cell counts and any of the psychosocial measures, but 62% of the sample had CD4+ counts below 100, thus restricting the range of observations. The critical factors of neurocognitive functioning, psychiatric history, and psychoactive drug use were not controlled in this study.

Psychological Well-Being

Although several of the above studies also included measures of psychological well-being, a few investigations have been more directly focused on psychological well-being. Studies of psychological well-being generally have been concerned with personal coping resources, defined as relatively stable dispositional characteristics (Moos & Schaefer, 1993), including such concepts as optimism/hope, sense of coherence, and hardiness.

Perhaps the best known research related to psychological well-being has been that of Solomon and associates with long-term survivors of AIDS. In a 1987 report of their pilot work, Solomon, Temoshok, O'Leary, and Zich compared 10 men who had died of *Pneumocystis carinii* pneumonia with 11 men who had survived that diagnosis. Although the long-term survivors used more problem-solving social support and had higher scores on the control dimension of Kobasa's (1979) hardiness measure, findings were confounded with time, in that the survivor group had been enrolled in the study for a considerably shorter period than had the unfavorable outcome group. In a 1993 letter to the editor, Solomon, Benton, Harker, Bonavida, and Fletcher reported their observations of normal NK cell cytotoxicity and frequent use of future-oriented, active coping strategies among nine gay men who had CD4+ cell counts of less than 50 and yet had been without HIV-related symptoms for an average of 19.2 months.

In a correlational study focused on the maintenance of hope among 124 HIV-infected gay men, Rabkin, Williams, Neugebauer, Remien, and Goetz (1990) found that hopelessness [using the Beck Hopelessness Scale (Beck, Weissman, Lester, & Trexler, 1974)] was negatively related to social support, positive-impact life events (on an adaptation of the Life Experiences Survey) internal locus of control, and commitment [measured by Kobasa's (1979) hardiness measure] and positively related to depression [indicated by clinical interviews based on the Hamilton scale (Williams, 1988)]. There were no significant relationships with HIV-related symptoms or CD4+ cell counts. However, potential PNI relationships were restricted, in that this group of participants had limited physical symptoms and, overall, high levels of hope and low levels of depression.

Among 94 HIV-infected individuals who were initially without AIDS, Solano et al. (1993) described psychosocial factors associated with HIV-disease progression. Baseline psychological scores reflecting lower fighting spirit and higher denial/repression were associated with the onset of AIDS-defining symptoms after 1 year. Less hardiness predicted lower CD4+ cell counts after 6 months, but there were no significant associations at 1 year among the immunological and psychosocial variables (including social support and loneliness, in addition to psychological attitudes and hardiness). However, immunological analyses were performed only for those subjects with baseline CD4+ cell counts above 300, resulting in restrictions of both the sample size ($n = 68$) and the range of variation for potentially correlated measures. The validity of the three-item measure of psychological attitudes used in this study is questionable. Additionally, the probability of type I errors was greatly increased by the use of excessive comparisons.

Nicholas and Webster (1993) examined relationships among hardiness, using the Health Related Hardiness Scale (Pollack & Dufty, 1990); social support, indicated by the Personal Resource Questionnaire (Weinert, 1987); and CD4+ T lymphocyte count among 46 HIV-infected men (15 of whom had self-reported AIDS) who were enrolled in support groups. Although there were no significant relationships with CD4+ cells, hardiness was directly related to social support. No controls for circadian pattern or other factors known to confound immune measures were reported. Design and analysis issues related to the combination of two nonequivalent participant groups, only one of which included stress management and nutrition education, confound interpretation of this study.

Interventions

PNI-related intervention studies with persons with HIV disease have thus far involved stress management approaches using cognitive-behavioral techniques or aerobic exercise training. Cognitive-behavioral stress management techniques are generally aimed at reducing psychological stress and enhancing coping skills to indirectly augment immune functioning. Goals of aerobic exercise training include reduction of anxiety and depression, increased release of endogenous opioids, and attenuation of autonomic nervous system responses to stress, which may indirectly and/or directly enhance immunity (LaPerriere, Antoni, et al., 1991; Schneiderman et al., 1994).

In one of the first published intervention studies, Coates, McKusick, Kuno, and Stites (1989) found that following an 8-week group stress management intervention with HIV-infected gay men ($N = 64$), there were no differences between the intervention and wait-list control groups in numbers of CD4$^+$ lymphocytes, the ratio of CD4$^+$ to CD8$^+$ cells, serum immunoglobulin A levels, NK cell cytotoxicity, or lymphocyte proliferative responses. Because controls for baseline CD4$^+$ cell levels, health status, and potential cofactors were only minimally described, the influences of such critical confounding factors as stage of illness, antiretroviral medications, and use of psychoactive substances cannot be adequately judged for this study.

Auerbach, Oleson, and Solomon (1992) conducted an intervention study in which 20 symptomatic gay males were randomly assigned to a wait-list or an 8-week training program in thermal biofeedback, guided imagery, and hypnosis. Intervention was associated with a decline in self-reported HIV symptomatology and increases in perceived vigor, as indicated by the Profile of Mood States, as well as hardiness, measured by the Kobasa scale. There were no significant findings in relation to CD4$^+$ cell counts or any of the psychological distress measures. Findings of this study are difficult to interpret because the timing of psychological measures in relation to CD4$^+$ cell counts, which were obtained from independent physician records, was not reported.

The preponderance of intervention research published to date has been conducted at the University of Miami's Center for the Biopsychosocial Study of AIDS. LaPerriere, Antoni, et al. (1991) and Schneiderman et al. (1994) have summarized this intervention research program, funded by the National Institute of Mental Health, which has thus far involved comparisons of 10-week programs of cognitive-behavioral stress management training or aerobic exercise training against randomized control groups. Subjects have been asymptomatic gay men, self-identified as being at risk for HIV infection, who were assessed by serial measures from 5 weeks before through 5 weeks after their first HIV-antibody test.

Although data were derived from subjects enrolled in intervention studies, two Miami publications were correlational reports focused on the concept of stress. Ironson et al. (1990) first reported changes associated with HIV-antibody testing. Six serial measures of psychological status and immunocompetence were obtained for 36 at-risk men over the 10 weeks surrounding HIV testing and for 25 laboratory control subjects who did not undergo testing. As expected, psychological distress levels, as indicated by the Impact of Event Scale (Horowitz et al., 1979), were higher postnotification for those subjects found to be HIV-seropositive, but no significant relationships between psychological distress and the immune measures were reported. In the HIV-seropositive group only, there was a relationship between increased anxiety on the State-Trait Anxiety Inventory (Spielberger, Gorsuch, Lushene, 1970) measured at the time of notification and decreased NK cell cytotoxicity measured 1 week later. There were no relationships between the seropositive group's higher anxiety at the time of notification and lymphocyte proliferation at any measurement occasion. Both NK cytotoxicity and psychological distress levels (including anxiety) returned to baseline values by 5 weeks postnotification. In this group of asymptomatic HIV-infected subjects, NK cell functioning appeared to be more responsive than lymphocyte proliferation to the acute stress surrounding HIV testing and serostatus notification.

Antoni, Schneiderman, et al. (1991) followed with a correlational report concerning neuroendocrine patterns during the week of serostatus notification among 25 HIV-seropositive and 46 seronegative men. The seropositive group had higher psychological distress, using a Profile of Mood States composite and the Impact of Event scale. Spot plasma cortisol values for HIV-seropositive subjects were lower than those for seronegative subjects at baseline and declined after notification, demonstrating inverse correlations between cortisol and concurrent measures of increased psychological distress. On the other hand, plasma cortisol was positively correlated with lymphocyte proliferation responses, although cortisol levels were significantly lower for HIV-seropositive subjects at all time points. This pattern was opposite to that of the HIV-seronegative group and contrary to PNI-predicted relationships, in that increased psychological distress would be expected to be accompanied by elevated cortisol and, in turn, decreased lymphocyte proliferation. Thus, the investigators suggested that dysregulation of the neuroendocrine and/or immune systems may account for disparities among psychological, neuroendocrine, and immunological measures in persons with HIV disease. These paradoxical findings also could be attributable to the inherent variability of one-time samples of plasma cortisol and may not be reflective of overall neuroendocrine functioning. The timing of the psychological and immune measures with respect to the stressor could account for additional variability in the observed data.

Within the same acute stress paradigm of HIV testing and serostatus notification at Miami, 47 gay men at risk for infection were randomly assigned to assessment-only control groups or cognitive-behavioral stress management groups that met twice weekly for 10 weeks. Antoni, Baggett, et al. (1991) found that over the 2-week pre- to postnotification period, HIV-seropositive intervention subjects had much lower depression scores on the Beck Depression Inventory and increased CD4+ and CD56+ counts in comparison to seropositive controls. There were no significant differences among groups in lymphocyte proliferative responses or in NK cell cytotoxicity, but among all subjects, pre- to postnotification changes in NK cell cytotoxicity were negatively correlated with anxiety. Among seropositive subjects in the stress management groups, frequency of relaxation practice was strongly associated with lower depression scores, higher CD4+ counts, and higher NK cell counts. Based on differences between the intervention and control groups, as well as relaxation practice effects, it is possible that cognitive-behavioral stress management buffered psychological distress associated with the acute stress of HIV testing and enhanced the selected quantitative immune measures. However, type I errors due to multiple univariate analyses (with small subgroup sizes) also could account for some of these findings.

LaPerriere et al. (1990) and LaPerriere, Fletcher, et al. (1991) tested the potential for aerobic exercise training to enhance immune functioning and reduce psychological distress within the Miami acute stress paradigm of HIV-serostatus testing. Asymptomatic but at-risk gay males were randomly assigned to assessment-only control groups or exercise training sessions conducted three times weekly for 10 weeks. Both seropositive and seronegative subjects in the exercise groups had significant increases in aerobic capacity by Week 5, which was maintained through the 10 weeks of training. Whereas seropositive control group subjects had significant increases in depression and anxiety using subscales of the Profile of Mood States and decreases in numbers of NK (CD56+) cells associated with HIV-serostatus notification, the seropositive exercise group did not show such changes. There were no significant changes in CD4+ cell counts or NK cell cytotoxicity for any of the groups. Thus, the quantitative measure of NK cells appeared to be adversely associated with psychological distress and responsive to aerobic exercise. The findings of both the Antoni, Baggett, et al. (1991) and LaPerriere group (1990) are somewhat surprising, in that other studies have indicated that functional immune measures may be more sensitive to psychological factors than are quantitative measures (Kiecolt-Glaser & Glaser, 1992). It may be that immune system dysfunction due to HIV disease masks interactions of psychological status and immune function measures, at least in some cases.

Esterling et al. (1992) reported the effects of both cognitive-behavioral stress management and aerobic exercise training on the modulation of Epstein-Barr virus (EBV) and herpes virus type-6 (HHV-6) antibodies over the 10-week serostatus testing period. Among 65 subjects, HIV-seropositive individuals had higher EBV antibody titers than those of seronegative subjects at all time points, indicating less immunological control of viral proliferation. There were no group differences in HHV-6 titers. Both HIV-seropositive and

HIV-seronegative subjects in both intervention groups had decreased antibody titers to EBV in comparison to their respective control groups, but changes in HHV-6 titers were not consistent. It may be that EBV (a predominantly B-cell pathogen) is more sensitive than HHV-6 (a virus that targets T cells) to psychosocial interventions. Additionally, the lack of serostatus-group differences in HHV-6 titers may reflect more effective immune system control of HHV-6, even in conjunction with immune system compromise.

Ironson et al. (1994) reported 1- and 2-year follow-up data for 23 of the Miami intervention and control group subjects. At 2 years after study entry, intervention per se was not correlated with disease progression. However, lower treatment adherence and participation as well as increased distress and denial following diagnosis were significantly associated with HIV-related symptoms and/or progression to AIDS.

Finally, Eller (1996) compared the cognitive-behavioral techniques of guided imagery and progressive muscle relaxation among 69 persons at various stages of HIV disease. Following the 6-week intervention delivered via audiotapes, the relaxation group had significantly less depression, using the Center for Epidemiological Studies–Depression Scale, and the guided imagery group had less fatigue, as indicated by the Sickness Impact Profile (Bergner, Bobbitt, Pollard, Martin, & Gilson, 1976). In comparison to the randomized control group, the relaxation group (only) had significantly higher postintervention CD4+ T lymphocyte counts, but there were no differences in numbers of NK (CD16+) cells for either treatment group. It is possible that stress induced by the virus-specific guided imagery script confounded the intervention effects and could account for the absence of immune modulation in that group.

Summary

Although data are limited and effect sizes are modest, there is general support for relationships between stress/coping patterns and clinical symptoms as well as immune measures in HIV-infected persons. Cumulative evidence has been limited by use of a variety of psychosocial stress measures, reliance on cell counts as immune system indicators, and a focus on gay men with early HIV disease.

In line with research with other populations (Herbert & Cohen, 1993a; Kemeny, Solomon, Morley, & Herbert, 1992; Weisse, 1992), there is some support for a relationship between psychological distress and immunity in persons with HIV disease. The largest cluster of studies has been focused on depressive symptomatology, but there remains controversy related to those data. Although in certain studies there is a relationship between psychological distress and physical symptoms, there have been no studies to provide knowledge of directionality (causality) in these relationships. Lack of significant relationships in many cases may be attributable to sample range restrictions, such as low levels of psychological distress or minimal immune system functioning. There have been few longitudinal studies, and in those cases in which longitudinal follow-up was attempted, data have been inconsistent. Stage of illness appears to be a critical variable over time.

Because there have been so few studies, which have concerned a variety of concepts, and some have had design and validity problems, there is as yet little support for relationships between psychological well-being and immunity. There also has been little attempt to examine psychological well-being in relation to clinical symptomatology.

Many of the intervention studies were correlational studies between stress or anxiety and immunity during the period of HIV testing and notification of serostatus. There is promising evidence that aerobic exercise and/or cognitive-behavioral therapies may improve immunity and/or delay symptoms and progression to AIDS. These interventions may serve as a buffer between anxiety at the time of diagnosis and altered immunity, but much more research is needed to document their potential influences on disease progression.

RESEARCH ISSUES AND
IMPLICATIONS FOR FUTURE RESEARCH

In the preceding pages, PNI studies involving HIV-infected subjects were individually reviewed with attention to major design and methodological issues. Additional, overriding issues concerning the difficulties involved in carrying out PNI research include those related to the measurement of stress, psychological status, and immune function; timing of research assessments; control of potential cofactors and confounding variables; and generalizability of findings.

PNI studies are fraught with methodological difficulties because of the multifactorial and complex nature of this type of research. At the initial meeting of what was to become the Psychoneuroimmunology Research Society in 1986, scientists grappled with the problem of how to define and measure stress (Cohen, 1987), an issue that has yet to be resolved. Physiological indices of stress are not often used in PNI research due to issues related to the construct validity of neuroendocrine-derived factors and the need to control for episodic bursts of hormones as a result of circadian periodicity or in response to bio-behavioral influences. Although multiple blood draws, salivary sampling, and 24-hour urine collections in part circumvent such issues, these approaches can be inconvenient, costly, and unreliable if not carefully designed and executed

(Kirschbaum & Hellhammer, 1992; Kuhn, 1989; Ziegler, 1989). In acute stress paradigms, recent technical advances have enhanced the measurement of autonomic responses as reflected by electrodermal and cardiovascular activity (Katkin, Dermit, & Wine, 1993). However, the measurement and interpretation of neuroendocrine parameters, particularly for studies of naturalistic and chronic stress, remain problematic (Kuhn, 1989; Ziegler, 1989).

For psychosocial stress measures, a major criticism continues to be the presumption of normative definitions of stressful life events (Derogatis & Coons, 1993), despite general agreement that the individual's subjective perception, or cognitive appraisal, is a critical determinant of the stress process (Folkman, 1993; Gorman & Kertzner, 1990). The most common measure of stress in studies with the HIV-infected population has been the Life Experiences Survey (Sarason, Johnson, & Siegel, 1978), which enables assessment of the personal valence of experienced stressors, thereby reducing criticism related to a normative approach. However, the Life Experiences Survey does not escape the related criticism that life events surveys may be irrelevant for the experiences of a given subgroup (Derogatis & Coons, 1993). With few exceptions (e.g., McCain & Cella, 1995; Reed et al., 1994), instrumentation for stress studies in persons with HIV disease have suffered from this critical problem. Interactional approaches for stress measurement [e.g., the Derogatis Stress Profile (Derogatis, 1980)] provide broader data on the stress process through integrated assessments of stimulus events, mediating variables, and response patterns (Derogatis & Coons, 1993). Issues about which little is yet known include the differences between acute and chronic psychological stress in terms of both the individual's perceptions and their differential influences on immunity and health (Gorman & Kertzner, 1990).

A central issue in the measurement of psychological distress, in general, is the confounding of dysphoric states with somatic symptoms. In the HIV literature in particular, psychological distress has been shown to be directly related to HIV symptomatology in several studies (e.g., Hayes, Turner, & Coates, 1992; Linn et al., 1993; Perry et al., 1992; van Servellen et al., 1993). With measures of psychological distress, items related to physical symptoms must be treated separately and/or omitted from analyses of immune parameters to avoid this source of confounding.

The selection of immune measures for study inclusion is largely dependent upon the research question and the nature of the study population. Although theory-driven selection of immune measures is often considered the most appropriate approach to follow (e.g., measuring cell-mediated immunity in cancer patients, quantifying levels of IgA in studies of respiratory viral infection), current knowledge of the linkages between immune aberrations and clinical outcomes is tenuous at best. It is possible that only large immunological changes will influence health status (Rabin et al., 1989). After selection of theoretically appropriate immune measure(s) for study, there remain issues of biological and analytical variability of the measures. To control assay variability, multiple baseline measures as well as replicate determinations at each research assessment are needed. For feasibility as well as for ethical reasons, many studies are carried out with immune cells obtained from peripheral venous blood samples, even though it is recognized that hormones such as cortisol may cause repopulation of peripheral blood cells to other immune organs (Fauci, 1975).

Further complicating the selection, measurement, and interpretation of immune parameters in HIV disease are the immunosuppressive effects of the virus and potential neuroendocrine dysregulation, both of which may affect immune reactivity to psychosocial factors (Antoni, Schneiderman, et al., 1991). Fundamental questions remain unanswered concerning PNI mechanisms in the context of an immune-mediated disease. For example, it has been recognized that persons who are immunosuppressed, such as the elderly, are more likely to experience further immunosuppression in response to psycho-social changes than are persons who have normal immune function (Targum, Marshall, Fischman, & Martin, 1989). On the other hand, it has been suggested that profound suppression of the immune system by HIV may create a floor effect such that no further reductions in immunological status could theoretically be observed (Kertzner, 1991). Exquisite research designs that account for baseline status and precise measures will be required to address these issues.

Although there continues to be controversy as to how best to define and measure stages of HIV illness and/or disease progression (Cohen, 1992), quantification of CD4[+] T lymphocytes remains the most frequently used indicator (Cohen, 1992; Stein et al., 1992). Also controversial is whether CD4[+] cell counts or percentages should be employed (Stein et al., 1992). Because HIV disease is marked by the destruction of CD4[+] T lymphocytes, the CD4[+] cell count historically has been the preferred biological indicator (Taylor, Fahey, Detels, & Giorgi, 1989), but measurement error related to calculation of the lymphocyte differential count must be considered. The CD4[+] percentage, which is directly obtained through flow-cytometric measurement (Centers for Disease Control [CDC], 1992a, 1992b; Fahey et al., 1990; Taylor et al., 1989), has been recommended by some investigators as the more reliable indicator for immunological assessments (e.g., Kessler, Landay, Pottage, & Benson, 1990; Taylor et al., 1989).

In view of the fact that CD4[+] T lymphocytes are rapidly replenished following destruction by HIV (Ho et al., 1995; Wei et al., 1995), CD4[+] cell levels may not be the best markers of disease activity, particularly when viral levels are relatively low. Other markers that have shown promise in predicting disease progression include β_2-microglobulin and neopterin (Fahey et al., 1990; Melmed et al., 1989; Schwartländer et al., 1993) and viral burden, as determined by newer methods such as quantitative competitive polymerase chain reaction and branched DNA signal-amplification assays (Cao, Qin, Zhang, Safrit, & Ho, 1995; Furtado, Murphy, & Wolinsky, 1993). Although investigators have thus far included few functional indicators of immune status, such measures as lymphocyte proliferation and NK cell cytotoxicity may be more sensitive to psychosocial factors than are quantitative measures (Kiecolt-Glaser & Glaser, 1992; Schulz & Schulz, 1992). Clearly, future studies will be enhanced by multiple measures of immune status.

In HIV studies, as in other PNI studies that involve persons with chronic illnesses, there are multiple issues concerning the timing of measures of stress and immune status. In addition to considerations of circadian fluctuations in neuroendocrine hormones and immune cells, researchers must account for the chronicity of the stress response and the timing of measurements in relation to stressful events (Stein & Miller, 1993). Furthermore, there are issues of repeated measures and patient follow-up for longitudinal studies. For example, evaluations of relevant immune system changes and, particularly, health outcomes require relatively long-term participant follow-up, perhaps years. Yet interval evaluations of psychosocial factors and concurrent immune measures also may be required every 3 to 6 months (Kemeny, 1994b). Critical questions remain for future investigators concerning the temporal relationships among perceived stress, psychological status, immune system effects, and health manifestations (Gorman & Kertzner, 1990).

PNI research is further complicated by numerous known and suspected cofactors and confounding variables, which present multiple issues that often have not been addressed or adequately controlled in past studies. Research controls through design strategies and statistical evaluation are needed for such variables as neuropsychological functioning, age, nutritional status, sleep patterns, physical activity, use of alcohol or psychoactive drugs, and menstrual phases. Of special concern in this area of research is confounding due to medications in general and antiretroviral drugs in particular. The use of immunomodulatory medications of all types must be controlled through matching strategies, statistical analysis, or participant exclusionary criteria (Kiecolt-Glaser & Glaser, 1988; Zeller, McCain, McCann, Swanson, & Colletti, in press).

For the most part, findings of studies to date have had quite limited generalizability. Whereas most PNI studies with the HIV population have thus far involved gay males, the nature of the epidemic is changing to include more women, adolescents, injection drug users, and racial/ethnic minorities (CDC, 1994). Earlier studies with gay males may not be generalizable to these subpopulations, as they are likely to experience different psychosocial stressors and altered disease trajectories and may exhibit changes in health behaviors that should be considered as confounding variables in the design and analysis of such studies.

CONCLUSION

Future PNI research with HIV-infected persons will benefit from prospective, longitudinal studies that include multiple measures of psychological, neuroendocrinological, immunological, and health status changes over time, as well as extensive data on extraneous variables. Because such studies are inherently multifactorial and complex, interdisciplinary consultation and/or research teams will be needed. Nurse scientists can be expected to add a unique perspective to PNI research by focusing on clinical care concerns with an aim to improve health outcomes.

Nursing research is making slow but steady progress in the area of HIV research. Prior to 1987 there were no research articles in the nursing literature (Larson, 1988). In 1988 the Conference on Research Priorities, convened by the National Institute of Nursing Research (NINR), identified HIV research as one of the institute's funding priorities. The priority expert panel that was assembled to focus this funding initiative identified the physiological and psychosocial aspects of nursing care as the major areas of emphasis (National Center for Nursing Research, 1990). As of June 1990, there had been 54 HIV-related research articles in the nursing literature; however, only 9 of these addressed physiological or psychological aspects of care, and none used a PNI framework to guide the investigation (Larson & Ropka, 1991).

At a subsequent NINR-sponsored Conference on Research Priorities in 1993, two related priorities were identified. The first specifically concerns HIV infection, with a focus on "assessing the effectiveness of nursing interventions in HIV/AIDS"; the second targets "identifying bio-behavioral factors and testing interventions to promote immunocompetence" ("Nurse Scientists," 1993, p. 1). These emphases are expected to encourage further research in the area of PNI as related to HIV disease. As evidenced by this review, six recent nursing studies of persons with HIV disease were based on an identifiable PNI framework to study HIV disease (Eller, 1996, Linn et al., 1993; McCain & Cella, 1995; Nicholas & Webster, 1993; Nokes & Kendrew, 1990; van Servellen et al., 1993). The uniqueness of these studies lies in their emphasis on life quality, which is critical when one considers that HIV infection is a devastating, chronic, debilitating disease that currently has no cure. From an interdisciplinary perspective, as well as nursing's holistic approach to caring, nursing science has much to offer in the rapidly developing interest area of PNI in HIV disease.

ACKNOWLEDGMENT

Dr. McCain was supported during the preparation of this manuscript by a postdoctoral fellowship from the National Institute of Nursing Research (T32 NR07052), Janice M. Zeller, PhD, RN, Program Director.

REFERENCES

Abbas, A. K., Lichtman, A. H., & Pober, J. S. (1994). *Cellular and molecular immunology* (2nd ed.). Philadelphia: Saunders.

Ader, R., Felton, D. L., & Cohen, N. (Eds.) (1991). *Psychoneuroimmunology* (2nd ed.). New York: Academic Press.

Antoni, M. H., Baggett, L., Ironson, G., LaPerriere, A., August, S., Klimas, N., Schneiderman, N., & Fletcher, M. A. (1991). Cognitive-behavioral stress management intervention buffers distress responses and immunologic changes following notification of HIV-1 seropositivity. *Journal of Consulting and Clinical Psychology, 59*, 906–915.

Antoni, M. H., Schneiderman, N., Fletcher, M. A., Goldstein, D. A., Ironson, G., & LaPerriere, A. (1990). Psychoneuroimmunology and HIV-1. *Journal of Consulting and Clinical Psychology, 58*, 38–49.

Antoni, M. H., Schneiderman, N., Klimas, N., LaPerriere, A., Ironson, G., & Fletcher, M. A. (1991). Disparities in psychological, neuroendocrine, and immunologic patterns in asymptomatic HIV-1 seropositive and seronegative gay men. *Biological Psychiatry, 29*, 1023–1041.

Auerbach, J. E., Oleson, T. D., & Solomon, G. F. (1992). A behavioral medicine intervention as an adjunctive treatment for HIV-related illness. *Psychology and Health, 6*, 325–334.

Barrett, D. C., Chesney, M. A., Burack, J. H., Stall, R. D., Ekstrand, M. L., & Coates, T. J. (1994). Depression and CD4 decline [Letter to the editor]. *Journal of the American Medical Association, 271*, 1743.

Beck, A. T., Ward, C. H., & Mendelson, M. (1961). An inventory for measuring depression. *Archives of General Psychiatry, 4*, 561–571.

Beck, A. T., Weissman, A., Lester, D., & Trexler, L. (1974). The measurement of pessimism: The Hopelessness Scale. *Journal of Consulting and Clinical Psychology, 42*, 861–865.

Bergner, M., Bobbitt, R. A., Pollard, W. E., Martin, D. P., & Gilson, B. S. (1976). *Medical Care, XIV*, 57–67.

Blalock, J. E. (1992). Production of peptide hormones and neurotransmitters by the immune system. In J. E. Blalock (Ed.), *Neuroimmunoendocrinology* (2nd rev. ed., (pp. 1–24). Basel, Switzerland: Karger.

Blaney, N. T., Goodkin, K., Feaster, D., Morgan, R., Baum, M., Wilkie, F., Szapocznik, J., & Eisdorfer, C. (1992). Life events and active coping style predict health status in early HIV-1 infection [Abstract]. *Proceedings of VIII International Conference on AIDS* (No. PuB 7215), *8*(PuB), 84.

Blaney, N. T., Goodkin, K., Morgan, R. O., Feaster, D., Millon, C., Szapocznik, J., & Eisdorfer, C. (1991). A stress-moderator model of distress in early HIV-1 infection: Concurrent analysis of life events, hardiness and social support. *Journal of Psychosomatic Research, 35*, 297–305.

Blatt, S. P., Hendrix, C. W., Butzin, C. A., Freeman, T. M., Ward, W. W., Hensley, R. E., Melcher, G. P., Donovan, D. J., & Boswell, R. N. (1993). Delayed-type hypersensitivity skin testing predicts progression to AIDS in HIV-infected patients. *Annals of Internal Medicine, 119,* 177–184.

Brenner. B. G., Dascal, A., Margolese, R. G., & Wainberg, M. A. (1989). Natural killer cell function in patients with acquired immunodeficiency syndrome and related diseases. *Journal of Leukocyte Biology, 46,* 75–83.

Burack, J. H., Barrett, D. C., Stall, R. D., Chesney, M. A., Ekstrand, M. L., & Coates, T. J. (1993). Depressive symptoms and CD4 lymphocyte decline among HIV-infected men. *Journal of the American Medical Association, 270,* 2568–2573.

Calabrese, J. R., Kling, M. A., & Gold, P. W. (1987). Alterations in immunocompetence during stress, bereavement, and depression: Focus on neuroendocrine regulation. *American Journal of Psychiatry, 144,* 1123–1134.

Cao, Y., Qin, L., Zhang, L., Safrit, J., & Ho, D. D. (1995). Virologic and immunologic characterization of long-term survivors of human immunodeficiency virus type 1 infection. *New England Journal of Medicine, 332,* 201–208.

Carver, C. S., Scheier, M. F., & Weintraub, J. K. (1989). Assessing coping strategies: A theoretically based approach. *Journal of Personality and Social Psychology, 56,* 267–283.

Cella, D. F. (1992). *Manual: Functional Assessment of Cancer Therapy (FACT) scales.* Chicago: Rush-Presbyterian-St. Luke's Medical Center.

Cella, D. F., Jacobsen, P. B., Orav, E. J., Holland, J. D., Silberfarb, P. M., & Rafla, S. (1987). A brief POMS measure of distress for cancer patients. *Journal of Chronic Diseases, 40,* 939–942.

Centers for Disease Control. (1992a). Guidelines for the performance of CD4$^+$ T-cell determinations in persons with human immunodeficiency virus infection. *Morbidity and Mortality Weekly Report, 41* (No. RR-8).

Centers for Disease Control. (1992b). 1993 revised classification system for HIV infection and expanded surveillance case definition for AIDS among adolescents and adults, 1993. *Morbidity and Mortality Weekly Report, 41* (No. RR-17).

Centers for Disease Control. (1994). Update: Impact of the expanded AIDS surveillance case definition for adolescents and adults on case reporting—United States, 1993. *Morbidity and Mortality Weekly Report, 43,* 160–161.

Clerici, M., Bevilacqua, M., Vago, T., Villa, M. L., Shearer, G. M., & Norbiato, G. (1994). An immunoendocrinological hypothesis of HIV infection. *Lancet, 343,* 1552–1553.

Clerici, M., & Shearer, G. M. (1993). A TH1→TH2 switch is a critical step in the etiology of HIV infection. *Immunology Today, 14,* 107–111.

Clerici, M., Stocks, N. I., Zajac, R. A., Boswell, R. N., Lucey, D. R., Via, C. S., & Shearer, G. M. (1989). Detection of three distinct patterns of T helper cell dysfunction in asymptomatic, human immunodeficiency virus-seropositive patients: Independence of CD4$^+$ cell numbers and clinical staging. *Journal of Clinical Investigation, 84,* 1892–1899.

Coates, T. J., McKusick, L., Kuno, R., & Stites, D. P. (1989). Stress reduction training changed number of sexual partners but not immune function in men with HIV. *American Journal of Public Health, 79,* 885–887.

Cohen, J. (1992). Searching for markers on the AIDS trail. *Science, 258,* 388–390.

Cohen, J. J. (1987). Methodological issues in behavioural immunology. *Immunology Today, 8,* 33–34.

Cohen, S., Tyrrell, D. A. J., & Smith, A. P. (1991). Psychological stress and suscep-tibility to the common cold. *New England Journal of Medicine, 325,* 606–612.

Cohen, S., & Williamson, G. M. (1991). Stress and infectious disease in humans. *Psychological Bulletin, 109,* 5–24.

Cooper, D. A., Tindall, B., Wilson, E. J., Imrie, A. A., & Penny, R. (1988). Character-ization of T lymphocyte responses during primary infection with human immu-nodeficiency virus. *Journal of Infectious Diseases, 157,* 889–896.

Derogatis, L. R. (1980). *The Derogatis Stress Profile (DSP).* Baltimore: Clinical Psy-chometric Research.

Derogatis. L. R.. & Coons, H. L. (1993). Self-report measures of stress. In L. Gold-berger & S. Breznitz (Eds.), *Handbook of stress: Theoretical and clinical as-pects* (2nd ed., pp. 200–233). New York: Free Press.

Derogatis, L. R., & Melisaratos, N. (1983). The Brief Symptom Inventory: An intro-ductory report. *Psychology and Medicine, 13,* 595–605.

Eller, L. S. (1996). Effects of two cognitive-behavioral interventions on immunity and symptoms in persons with HIV. *Annals of Behavioral Medicine, 17,* 339–348.

Esterling, B. A., Antoni, M. H., Schneiderman, N., Carver, C. S., LaPerriere, A., Ironson, G., Klimas, N. G., & Fletcher, M. A. (1992). Psychosocial modulation of antibody to Epstein-Barr viral capsid antigen and human herpes virus type-6 in HIV-1–infected and at-risk gay men. *Psychosomatic Medicine, 54,* 354–371.

Evans, D. L., Leserman, J., Perkins, D. O., Murphy, C., & Folds, J. D. (1992). Rela-tionship of social support and immunity in HIV [Abstract]. *Proceedings of VIII International Conference on AIDS* (No. PoC 4384), 8(PoC), C309.

Evans, D. L., Leserman, J., Perkins, D. O., Stern, R. A., Van der horst, C. M., Hall, C. D., & Folds, J. D. (1991). Stress related reduction of natural killer cells in HIV [Abstract]. *Proceedings of VII International Conference on AIDS* (No. ThB 91), 7(ThB), 79.

Fahey, J. L., Taylor, J. M. G., Detels, R., Hofmann, B., Melmed, R., Nishanian, P., & Giorgi, J. V. (1990). The prognostic value of cellular and serologic markers in infection with human immunodeficiency virus type 1. *New England Journal of Medicine, 322,* 166–172.

Fauci, A. S. (1975). Mechanisms of corticosteroid action on lymphocyte subpopula-tions: 1. Redistribution of circulating T and B lymphocytes to the bone mar-row. *Immunology, 28,* 669–680.

Folkman, S. (1993). Psychosocial effects of HIV infection. In L. Goldberger & S. Breznitz (Eds.), *Handbook of stress: Theoretical and clinical aspects* (pp. 658–681). New York: Free Press.

Folkman, S., & Lazarus, R. S. (1980). An analysis of coping in a middle-aged com-munity sample. *Journal of Health and Social Behavior, 21,* 219–239.

Furtado, M. R., Murphy, R., & Wolinsky, S. M. (1993). Quantification of human immunodeficiency virus type 1 tat mRNA as a marker for assessing the effi-cacy of antiretroviral therapy. *Journal of Infectious Diseases, 167,* 213–216.

Gartner, S., Markovits, P., Markovitz, D. M., Kaplan, M. H., Gallo, R. C., & Popovic, M. (1986). The role of mononuclear phagocytes in HTLV-III/LAV infection. *Science, 233,* 215–218.

Gendelman, H. E., & Meltzer, M. S. (1989). HIV-infected monocytes in the patho-genesis of AIDS. In M. Zembala & G. L. Asherston (Eds.), *Human monocytes* (pp. 469–481). London: Academic Press.

Glaser, R., & Kiecolt-Glaser, J. (1987). Stress-associated depression in cellular immunity: Implications for acquired immune deficiency syndrome (AIDS). *Brain, Behavior, and Immunity*, 1, 107–112.

Glaser, R., Pearson, G. R., Jones, J. F., Hillhouse, J., Kennedy, S., Mao, H., & Kiecolt-Glaser, J. K. (1991). Stress-related activation of Epstein-Barr virus. *Brain, Behavior, and Immunity*, 5, 219–232.

Glaser, R., Rice, J., Sheridan, J., Fertel, R., Stout, J., Speicher, C., Pinsky, D., Kotur, M., Post, A., Beck. M., & Kiecolt-Glaser, J. (1987). Stress-related immune suppression: Health implications. *Brain, Behavior, and Immunity*, 1, 7–20.

Goodkin, K., Blaney, N. T., Feaster, D., Fletcher, M. A., Baum, M. K., Mantero-Atienza, E., Klimas, N. G., Millon, C., Szapocznik, J., & Eisdorfer, C. (1992). Active coping style is associated with natural killer cell cytotoxicity in asymptomatic HIV-1 seropositive homosexual men. *Journal of Psychosomatic Research*, 36, 635–650.

Goodkin, K., Blaney, N., Feaster, D., Klimas, N., Fletcher, M. A., & Baum, M. (1993). Psychosocial variables predict long-term changes in psychological distress and laboratory progression markers of HIV-1 infection [Abstract]. *Proceedings of IX International Conference on AIDS* (No. PoD22–4074), 9(PoD), 897.

Goodkin, K., Fuchs, I., Feaster, D., Leeka, J., & Rishel, D. D. (1992). Life stressors and coping style are associated with immune measures in HIV-1 infection: A preliminary report. *International Journal of Psychiatry in Medicine*, 22, 155–172.

Gorman, J. M., & Kertzner, R. (1990). Psychoneuroimmunology and HIV infection. *Journal of Neuropsychiatry*, 2, 241–252.

Gorman, J. M., Kertzner, R., Cooper, T., Goetz, R. R., Lagomasino, I., Novacenko, H., Williams, J. B. W., Stern, Y., Mayeux, R., & Ehrhardt, A. A. (1991). Glucocorticoid level and neuropsychiatric symptoms in homosexual men with HIV infection. *American Journal of Psychiatry*, 148, 41–45.

Gruen, R. J. (1993). Stress and depression: Toward the development of integrative models. In L. Goldberger & S. Breznitz (Eds.), *Handbook of stress: Theoretical and clinical aspects* (2nd ed., pp. 550–569). New York: Free Press.

Guenter, P., Muurahainen, N., Simons, G., Kosok, A., Cohan, G. R., Rudenstein, R., & Turner, J. L. (1993). Relationships among nutritional status, disease progression, and survival in HIV infection. *Journal of Acquired Immune Deficiency Syndromes*, 6, 1130–1138.

Hayes, R. B., Turner, H., & Coates, T. J. (1992). Social support, AIDS-related symptoms, and depression among gay men. *Journal of Consulting and Clinical Psychology*, 60, 463–469.

Herbert, T. B., & Cohen, S. (1993a). Depression and immunity: A meta-analytic review. *Psychological Bulletin*, 113, 472–486.

Herbert, T. B., & Cohen, S. (1993b). Stress and immunity in humans: A meta-analytic review. *Psychosomatic Medicine*, 55, 364–379.

Herzberg, U., Murtaugh, M., & Beitz, A. J. (1994). Chronic pain and immunity: Mononeuropathy alters immune responses in rats. *Pain*, 59, 219–225.

Ho, D. D., Neumann, A. U., Perelson, A. S., Chen, W., Leonard, J. M., & Markowitz, M. (1995). Rapid turnover of plasma virions and CD4 lymphocytes in HIV-1 infection. *Nature*, 373, 123–126.

Horowitz, M., Wilner, N., & Alvarez, W. (1979). Impact of Event Scale: A measure of subjective stress. *Psychosomatic Medicine*, 41, 209–218.

Hulstaert, F., Strauss, K., Levacher, M., Vanham, G., Kestens, L., & Bach, B. A. (1992). The staging and prognostic value of subset markers in CD8 cells in HIV disease. In G. Jannossy, B. Autran, & F. Miedema (Eds.), *Immunodeficiency in HIV infection and AIDS: EC/FERS/MRC workshop on immunodeficiency in HIV-1 infections, Windsor, Surrey,* 1991 (pp. 185–194). Basel, Switzerland: Karger.

Ironson, G., Friedman, A., Klimas, N., Antoni, M., Fletcher, M. A., LaPerriere, A., Simoneau, J., & Schneiderman, N. (1994). Distress, denial, and low adherence to behavioral interventions predict faster disease progression in gay men infected with human immunodeficiency virus. *International Journal of Behavioral Medicine, 1,* 90–105.

Ironson, G., LaPerriere, A., Antoni, M., O'Hearn, P., Schneiderman, N., Klimas, N., & Fletcher, M. A. (1990). Changes in immune and psychological measures as a function of anticipation and reaction to news of HIV-1 antibody status. *Psychosomatic Medicine, 52,* 247–270.

Katkin, E. S., Dermit, S., & Wine, S. K. F. (1993). Psychophysiological assessment of stress. In L. Goldberger & S. Breznitz (Eds.), *Handbook of stress: Theoretical and clinical aspects* (2nd ed., pp. 142–157). New York: Free Press.

Kemeny, M. E. (1994a). Psychoneuroimmunology of HIV infection. *Psychiatric Clinics of North America, 17*(1), 55–68.

Kemeny, M. E. (1994b). Stressful events, psychological responses, and progression of HIV infection. In J. K. Kiecolt-Glaser & R. Glaser (Eds.), *Handbook of human stress and immunity* (pp. 245–266). San Diego: Academic Press.

Kemeny, M. E., Solomon, G. F., Morley, J. E., & Herbert, T. L. (1992). Psychoneuroimmunology. In C. B. Nemeroff (Ed.), *Neuroendocrinology* (pp. 563–591). Boca Raton, FL: CRC Press.

Kemeny, M. E., Weiner, H., Taylor, S. E., Schneider, S., Visscher, B., & Fahey, J. L. (1994). Repeated bereavement, depressed mood, and immune parameters in HIV seropositive and seronegative gay men. *Health Psychology, 13,* 14–24.

Kertzner, R. M. (1991). Future directions for psychoimmunology: HIV infection and beyond. In J. M. Gorman & R. M. Kertzner (Eds.), *Psychoimmunology update* (pp. 153–163). Washington, DC: American Psychiatric Press.

Kertzner, R. M., Goetz, R., Todak, G., Cooper, T., Lin, S. H., Reddy, M. M., Novacenko, H., Williams, J. B. W., Ehrhardt, A. A., & Gorman, J. M. (1993). Cortisol levels, immune status, and mood in homosexual men with and without HIV infection. *American Journal of Psychiatry, 150,* 1674–1678.

Kessler, H. A., Landay, A., Pottage, J. C., & Benson, C. A. (1990). Absolute number versus percentage of T-helper lymphocytes in human immunodeficiency virus infection. *Journal of Infectious Diseases, 161,* 356–357.

Kessler, R. C., Foster, C., Joseph, J., Ostrow, D., Wortman, C., Phair, J., & Chmiel, J. (1991). Stressful life events and symptom onset in HIV infection. *American Journal of Psychiatry, 148,* 733–738.

Khansari, D. N., Murgo, A. J., & Faith, R. E. (1990). Effects of stress on the immune system. *Immunology Today, 11,* 170–175.

Kiecolt-Glaser, J. K., Dura, J. R., Speicher, C. E., Trask, O. J., & Glaser, R. (1991). Spousal caregivers of dementia victims: Longitudinal changes in immunity and health. *Psychosomatic Medicine, 53,* 345–362.

Kiecolt-Glaser, J. K., Fisher, L. D., Ogrocki, P., Stout, J. C., Speicher, C. E., & Glaser, R. (1987). Marital quality, marital disruption, and immune function. *Psychosomatic Medicine, 49,* 13–34.

Kiecolt-Glaser, J. K., & Glaser, R. (1988). Methodological issues in behavioral immunology research with humans. *Brain, Behavior, and Immunity, 2,* 67–78.

Kiecolt-Glaser, J. K., & Glaser, R. (1992). Psychoneuroimmunology: Can psychological interventions modulate immunity? *Journal of Consulting and Clinical Psychology*, *60*, 569–575.

Kiecolt-Glaser, J. K., & Glaser, R. (Eds.) (1994). *Handbook of human stress and immunity*. San Diego: Academic Press.

Kirschbaum, C., & Hellhammer, D. (1992). Methodological aspects of salivary cortisol measurement. In C. Kirschbaum, G. F. Read, & D. H. Hellhammer (Eds.), *Assessment of hormones and drugs in saliva in biobehavioral research* (pp. 19–32). Seattle: Hogrefe & Huber.

Kobasa, S. (1979). Stressful life events, personality, and health: An inquiry into hardiness. *Journal of Personality and Social Psychology*, *37*, 1–11.

Koenig, S., Gendelman, H. E., Orenstein, J. M., DalCanto, M. C., Pezeshkpour, G. H., Yungbluth, M., Janotta, F., Aksamit, A., Martin, M. A., & Fauci, A. S. (1986). Detection of AIDS virus in macrophages in brain tissue from AIDS patients with encephalopathy. *Science*, *233*, 1089–1093.

Kolesnitchenko, V., & Snart, S. (1992). Regulatory elements in the human immunodeficiency virus type 1 long terminal repeat LTR (HIV-1) responsive to steroid hormone stimulation. *AIDS Research and Human Retroviruses*, *8*, 1977–1980.

Kuby, J. (1994). *Immunology* (2nd ed.). New York: Freeman.

Kuhn, C. M. (1989). Adrenocortical and gonadal steroids in behavioral cardiovascular medicine. In N. Schneiderman, S. M. Weiss, & P. G. Kaufmann (Eds.), *Handbook of research methods in cardiovascular behavioral medicine* (pp. 185–204). New York: Plenum.

Lane, H. C., Masur, H., Edgar, L. C., Whalen, G., Rook, A. H., & Fauci, A. S. (1983). Abnormalities of B-cell activation and immunoregulation in patients with the acquired immunodeficiency syndrome. *New England Journal of Medicine*, *309*, 453–458.

Lang, W., Perkins, H., Anderson, R. E., Royce, R., Jewell, N., & Winkelstein, W. (1989). Patterns of T lymphocyte changes with human immunodeficiency virus infection: From seroconversion to the development of AIDS. *Journal of Acquired Immune Deficiency Syndromes*, *2*, 63–69.

LaPerriere, A., Antoni, M., Klimas, N., Ironside, G., Schneiderman, N., & Fletcher, M. A. (1991). Psychoimmunology and stress management in HIV-1 infection. In J. M. Gorman & R. M. Kertzner (Eds.), *Psychoimmunology update* (pp. 81–112). Washington, DC: American Psychiatric Press.

LaPerriere, A. R., Antoni, M. H., Schneiderman, N., Ironson, G., Klimas, N., Caralis, P., & Fletcher, M. A. (1990). Exercise intervention attenuates emotional distress and natural killer cell decrements following notification of positive serologic status for HIV-1. *Biofeedback and Self-Regulation*, *15*, 229–242.

LaPerriere, A., Fletcher, M. A., Antoni, M. H., Klimas, N. G., Ironson, G., & Schneiderman, N. (1991). Aerobic exercise training in an AIDS risk group. *International Journal of Sports Medicine*, *12*(Suppl. 1), S53–S57.

Larson, E. (1988). Nursing research and AIDS. *Nursing Research*, *37*, 60–62.

Larson, E., & Ropka, M. E. (1991). An update on nursing research and HIV infection. *Image: Journal of Nursing Scholarship*, *23*, 4–12.

Levy, J. A. (1994). Long-term survivors of HIV infection. *Hospital Practice*, *29*(10), 41–52.

Levy, S. M., Herberman, R. B., Maluish, A. M., Schlien, B., & Lippman, M. (1985). Prognostic risk assessment in primary breast cancer by behavioral and immunological parameters. *Health Pychology*, *4*, 99–113.

Lewis, F., Firsich, S., & Parsell, S. (1979). Clinical tool development for adult chemo-therapy patients: Process and content. *Cancer Nursing, 2,* 99–108.

Lewis, F., & Gallison, M. (1989). *Family functioning study* (Technical paper). Seattle: University of Washington.

Linn, J. G., Monnig, R. L., Cain, V. A., & Usoh, D. (1993). Stage of illness, level of HIV symptoms, sense of coherence and psychological functioning in clients of community-based AIDS counseling centers. *Journal of the Association of Nurses in AIDS Care, 4*(2), 24–32.

Livingston, I. L. (1988). Co-factors, host susceptibility, and AIDS: An argument for stress. *Journal of the National Medical Association, 80,* 49–59.

Lyketsos, C. G., Hoover, D., & Guccione, M. (1994). In reply [to Barrett et al., Letter to editor]. *Journal of the American Medical Association, 271,* 1743–1744.

Lyketsos, C. G., Hoover, D. K., Guccione, M., Senterfitt, W., Dew, M. A., Wesch, J., VanRaden, M. J., Treisman, G. J., & Morgenstern, H., for the Multicenter AIDS Cohort Study. (1993). Depressive symptoms as predictors of medical outcomes in HIV infection. *Journal of the American Medical Association, 270,* 2563–2567.

MacDonnell, K. B., Chmiel, J. S., Poggensee, L., Wu, S., & Phair, J. P. (1990). Pre-dicting progression to AIDS: Combined usefulness of CD4 lymphocyte counts and p24 antigenemia. *American Journal of Medicine, 89,* 706–712.

McCain, N. L., & Cella, D. F. (1995). Correlates of stress in HIV disease. *Western Journal of Nursing Research, 17,* 141–155.

McCain, N. L., & Gramling, L. F. (1992). Living with dying: Coping with HIV dis-ease. *Issues in Mental Health Nursing, 13,* 271–284.

McNair, D. M., Lorr, M., & Droppleman, L. F. (1971). *Edits manual: Profile of Mood States.* San Diego: Educational and Industrial Testing Service.

Melmed, R. N., Taylor, J. M. G., Bozorgmehri, M., & Fahey, J. L. (1989). Serum neopterin changes in HIV-infected subjects: Indicator of significant pathology, CD4 T cell changes, and the development of AIDS. *Journal of Acquired Im-mune Deficiency Syndromes, 1,* 70–76.

Miedema, F., Tersmette, M., & van Lier, R. A. W. (1990). AIDS pathogenesis: A dynamic interaction between HIV and the immune system. *Immunology Today, 11,* 293–297.

Migliorati, G., Nicoletti, I., D'Adamio, F., Spreca, A., Pagliacci, C., & Riccardi, C. (1994). Dexamethasone induces apoptosis in mouse natural killer cells and cyto-toxic T lymphocytes. *Immunology, 81,* 21–26.

Millon, T., Green, C., & Meagher, R. (1982). *Millon Behavioral Health Inventory manual.* Minneapolis: National Computer Services.

Mishel, M. H. (1981). The measurement of uncertainty in illness. *Nursing Research, 30,* 258–263.

Mishel, M. H. (1984). Perceived uncertainty and stress in illness. *Research in Nurs-ing and Health, 7,* 163–171.

Moos, R. H., & Schaefer, J. A. (1993). Coping resources and processes: Current con-cepts and measures. In L. Goldberger & S. Breznitz (Eds.), *Handbook of stress: Theoretical and clinical aspects* (2nd ed, pp. 234–257). New York: Free Press.

Mulder, C. L., & Antoni, M. H. (1992). Psychosocial correlates of immune status and disease progression in HIV-1 infected homosexual men: Review of preliminary findings, and commentary. *Psychology and Health, 6,* 175–192.

Namir, S., Wolcott, D. L., Fawzy, F. I., & Alumbaugh. M. J. (1987). Coping with AIDS: Psychological and health implications. *Journal of Applied Social Psy-chology 17,* 309–328.

National Center for Nursing Research. (1990). *HIV infection: Prevention and care: A report of the NCNR priority expert panel on HIV infection.* Bethesda, MD: Author.

Newberry, B. H., Jaikins-Madden, J. E., & Gerstenberger, T. J. (1991). *A holistic conceptualization of stress and disease.* New York: AMS Press.

Nicholas, P. K., & Webster, A. (1993). Hardiness and social support in human immunodeficiency virus. *Applied Nursing Research, 6,* 132–136.

Nicholson, J. K. A., Cross, G. D., Callaway, C. S., & McDougal, J. S. (1986). In vitro infection of human monocytes with human T lymphotropic virus type III/lymphadenopathy-associated virus (HTLVIII/LAV).*Journal of Immunology, 137,* 323–329.

Nokes, K. M., & Kendrew, J. (1990). Loneliness in veterans with AIDS and its relationship to the development of infections.*Archives of Psychiatric Nursing, 4,* 271–277.

Nurse scientists set research agenda to the year 2000. (1993).*NCNR Outreach,* Spring, pp. 1, 8.

O'Leary, A. (1990). Stress, emotion, and human immune function. *Psychological Bulletin, 108,* 363–382.

Palmblad, J., Petrini, B., Wasserman, J., & Åkerstedt, T. (1979). Lymphocyte and granulocyte reactions during sleep deprivation.*Psychosomatic Medicine, 41,* 273–278.

Pauza, C. D. (1988). HIV persistence in monocytes leads to pathogenesis and AIDS. *Cellular Immunology, 112,* 414–424.

Perry, S., & Fishman, B. (1993). Depression and HIV: How does one affect the other? [Editorial]. *Journal of the American Medical Association, 270,* 2609–2610.

Perry, S., Fishman, B., Jacobsberg, L., & Frances, A. (1992). Relationships over 1 year between lymphocyte subsets and psychosocial variables among adults with infection by human immunodeficiency virus. *Archives of General Psychiatry, 49,* 396–401.

Piatak, M., Saag, M. S., Yang, L. C., Clark, S. J., Kappes, J. C., Luk, K. C., Hahn, B. H., Shaw, G. M., & Lifson. J. D. (1993). High levels of HIV-1 in plasma during all stages of infection determined by competitive PCR. *Science, 259,* 1749–1754.

Plotnikoff, N., Murgo, A., Faith, R., & Wybran, J. (Eds.). (1991). *Stress and immunity.* Boca Raton, FL: CRC Press.

Pollock, S. E., & Duffy, M. E. (1990). The Health-Related Hardiness Scale: Development and psychometric analysis. *Nursing Research, 39,* 218–222.

Rabin, B. S., Cohen, S., Ganguli, R., Lysle, D. T., & Cunnick, J. E. (1989). Bidirectional interaction between the central nervous system and the immune system. *Critical Reviews in Immunology, 9,* 279–312.

Rabkin, J. G., Williams, J. B. W., Neugebauer, R., Remien, R. H., & Goetz, R. (1990). Maintenance of hope in HIV-spectrum homosexual men. *American Journal of Psychiatry, 147,* 1322–1326.

Rabkin, J. G., Williams, J. B. W., Ramien, R. H., Goetz, R., Kertzner, R., & Gorman, J. M. (1991). Depression, distress, lymphocyte subsets, and human immunodeficiency virus symptoms on two occasions in HIV-positive homosexual men. *Archives of General Psvchiatry, 48,* 111–119.

Radloff, L. S. (1977). The CES-D scale: A self-report depression scale for research in the general population. *Applied Psychological Measurement, 1,* 385–401.

Reed, G. M., Kemeny, M. E., Taylor, S. E., Wang, H. Y. J., & Visscher, B. R. (1994). Realistic acceptance as a predictor of decreased survival time in gay men with AIDS. *Health Psychology, 13,* 299–307.

Reichlin, S. (1993). Neuroendocrine-immune interactions. *New England Journal of Medicine, 329*, 1246–1252.

Robertson, K. R., Wilkins, J. W., Handy, J., van der Horst, C., Robertson, W. T., Fryer, J. G., Evans, D., & Hall, C. D. (1993). Psychoimmunology and AIDS: Psychological distress and herpes simplex virus in human immunodeficiency virus infected individuals. *Psychology and Health, 8*, 317–327.

Roitt, I., Brostoff, J., & Male, D. (1993). *Immunology* (3rd ed.). London: Mosby.

Roy, S., & Wainberg, M. A. (1988). Role of the mononuclear phagocyte system in the development of acquired immunodeficiency syndrome (AIDS). *Journal of Leukocyte Biology, 43*, 91–97.

Sahs, J. A., Goetz, R., Reddy, M., Rabkin, J. G., Williams, J. B. W., Kertzner, R., & Gorman, J. M. (1994). Psychological distress and natural killer cells in gay men with and without HIV infection. *American Journal of Psychiatry, 151*, 1479–1484.

Sarason, I. G., Johnson, J. H., & Siegel, J. M. (1978). Assessing the impact of life changes: Development of the Life Experiences Survey. *Journal of Consulting and Clinical Psychology, 46*, 932–946.

Sarason, I., Sarason, B., Potter, E., & Antoni, M. (1985). Life events, social support and illness. *Psychosomatic Medicine, 47*, 156–163.

Sarason, I., Sarason, B., Shearin, E. N., & Pierce, G. R (1987). A brief measure of social support: Practical and theoretical implications. *Journal of Social and Personal Relationships, 4*, 497–510.

Schleifer, S. J., Keller, S. E., Bond, R. N., Cohen, J., & Stein, M. (1989). Major depressive disorder and immunity: Role of age, sex, severity, and hospitalization. *Archives of General Psychiatry, 46*, 81–87.

Schmidt, N., & Sermat, V. (1983). Measuring loneliness in different relationships. *Journal of Personality and Social Psychology, 44*, 1038–1047.

Schneiderman, N., Antoni, M. H., Fletcher, M. A., Ironson, G., Klimas, N., Kumar, M., & LaPerriere, A. (1993). Stress, endocrine responses, immunity and HIV-1 spectrum disease. In H. Friedman, T. W. Klein, & S. Specter (Eds.), *Drugs of abuse, immunity, and AIDS* (pp. 225–234). New York: Plenum Press.

Schneiderman, N., Antoni, M., Ironson, G., Klimas, N., LaPerriere, A., Kumar, M., Esterling, B., & Fletcher, M. A. (1994). HIV-1, immunity, and behavior. In R. Glaser & J. Kiecolt-Glaser (Eds.), *Handbook of human stress and immunity* (pp. 267–300). San Diego: Academic Press.

Schnittman, S. M., Greenhouse, J. J., Psallidopoulos, M. C., Baseler, M., Salzman, N. P., Fauci, A. S., & Lane, H. C. (1990). Increasing viral burden in CD4+ T cells from patients with human immunodeficiency virus (HIV) infection reflects rapidly progressive immunosuppression and clinical disease. *Annals of Internal Medicine, 113*, 438–443.

Schulz, K. H., & Schulz. H. (1992). Overview of psychoneuroimmunological stress and intervention studies in humans with emphasis on the uses of immunological parameters. *Psycho-oncology, 1*, 51–70.

Schwartländer, B., Bek, B., Skarabis, H., & Koch, M. A. for the Multicentre Cohort Study Group. (1993). Improvement of the predictive value of CD4+ lymphocyte count by β_2-microglobulin, immunoglobulin A and erythrocyte sedimentation rate. *AIDS, 7*, 813–821.

Shearer, G. M., & Clerici, M. (1992). T helper cell immune dysfunction in asymptomatic, HIV-1-seropositive individuals: The role of TH1-TH2 cross-regulation. In R. L. Coffman (Ed.), *Chemical immunology: Vol. 54. Regulation and functional significance of T-cell subsets* (pp. 21–43). Basel, Switzerland: Karger.

Solano, L., Costa, M., Salvati, S., Coda, R., Aiuti, F., Mezzaroma, I., & Bertini, M. (1993). Psychosocial factors and clinical evolution in HIV-1 infection: A longitudinal study. *Journal of Psychosomatic Research, 37,* 39–51.

Solomon, G. F. (1987). Psychoneuroimmunologic approaches to research on AIDS. *Annals of the New York Academy of Sciences, 496,* 628–636.

Solomon, G. F., Benton. D., Harker, J. O., Bonavida, B., & Fletcher, M. A. (1993). Prolonged asymptomatic states in HIV-seropositive persons with 50 CD4+ T-cells/mm³: Preliminary psychoimmunologic findings [Letter to the editor]. *Journal of Acquired Immune Deficiency Syndromes, 6,* 1172.

Solomon. G. F., Kemeny, M. E., & Temoshok, L. (1991). Psychoneuroimmunologic aspects of human immunodeficiency virus infection. In R. Ader, D. L. Felton, & N. Cohen (Eds.), *Psychoneuroimmunology* (2nd ed., pp. 1081–1113). New York: Academic Press.

Solomon, G. F., & Temoshok, L. (1987). A psychoneuroimmunologic perspective on AIDS research: Questions, preliminary findings, and suggestions. *Journal of Applied Social Psychology, 17,* 286–308.

Solomon, G. F., Temoshok, L., O'Leary, A., & Zich, J. (1987). An intensive psychoimmunologic study of long-surviving persons with AIDS. *Annals of the New York Academy of Sciences, 496,* 647–655.

Spielberger, C., Gorsuch, R., & Lushene (1970). *State-Trait Anxiety Inventory manual.* Palo Alto, CA: Consulting Psychologists Press.

Stein, D. S., Korvick, J. A., & Vermund, S. T. (1992). CD4+ lymphocyte cell enumeration for prediction of clinical course of human immunodeficiency virus disease: A review. *Journal of Infectious Diseases, 165,* 352–363.

Stein, M., & Miller, A. H. (1993). Stress, the immune system, and health and illness. In L. Goldberger & S. Breznitz (Eds.), *Handbook of stress: Theoretical and clinical aspects* (2nd ed., pp. 127–141). New York: Free Press.

Stevenson, M., Stanwick, T. L., Dempsey, M. P., & Lamonica, C. A. (1990). HIV-1 replication is controlled at the level of T cell activation and proviral integration. *EMBO Journal, 9,* 1551–1560.

Stoner, M. (1982). Hope and cancer patients. *Dissertation Abstracts International, 43,* 1983B. (Univesity Microfilms No. 83-12, 243).

Strawn, J. M. (1991). The psychosocial consequences of HIV infection. In J. D. Durham, & F. L. Cohen (Eds.), *The person with AIDS: Nursing perspectives* (2nd ed., pp. 113–134). New York: Springer Publishing Co.

Targum, S. D., Marshall, L. E., Fischman, P., & Martin, D. (1989). Lymphocyte subpopulations in depressed elderly women. *Biological Psychiatry, 26,* 581–589.

Taylor, J. M. G., Fahey, J. L., Detels, R., & Giorgi, J. V. (1989). CD4 percentage, CD4 number, and CD4:CD8 ratio in HIV infection: Which to choose and how to use. *Journal of Acquired Immune Deficiency Syndromes, 2,* 114–124.

Taylor, R. (1994). Histocompatibility antigens, protective immunity, and HIV-1. *Journal of NIH Research, 6,* 68–71.

van Servellen, G., Padilla, G., Brecht, M. L., & Knoll, L. (1993). The relationship of stressful life events, health status and stress-resistance resources in persons with AIDS. *Journal of the Association of Nurses in AIDS Care, 4*(1), 11–22.

Watret, K. C., Whitelaw, J. A., Froebel, K. S., & Bird, A. G. (1993). Phenotypic characterization of CD8+ T cell populations in HIV disease and anti-HIV immunity. *Clinical and Experimental Immunology, 92,* 93–99.

Wei, X., Ghosh, S. K., Taylor, M. E., Johnson, V. A., Emini, E. A., Deutsch, P., Lifson,

J. D., Bonhoeffer, S., Nowak, M. A., Hahn, B. H., Saag, M. S., & Shaw, G. M. (1995). Viral dynamics in human immunodeficiency virus type 1 infection. *Nature, 373,* 117–122.

Weinert, C. (1987). A social support measure: PRQ85. *Nursing Research, 36,* 273–277.

Weiss, R. A. (1993). How does HIV cause AIDS? *Science, 260,* 1273–1279.

Weisse, C. S. (1992). Depression and immunocompetence: A review of the literature. *Psychological Bulletin, 111,* 475–489.

Williams, J. B. W. (1988). A structured interview guide for the Hamilton depression scale. *Archives of General Psychiatry, 45,* 742–747.

Zack, J. A., Arrigo, S. J., Weitsman, S. R., Go, A. S., Haislip, A., & Chen, I. S. Y. (1990). HIV-1 entry into quiescent primary lymphocytes: Molecular analysis reveals a labile, latent viral structure. *Cell, 61,* 213–222.

Zeller, J. M., McCain, N. L., McCann, J. J., Swanson, B., & Colletti, M. A. (in press). Methodological issues in psychoneuroimmunology research. *Nursing Research.*

Ziegler, M. G. (1989). Catecholamine measurement in behavioral research. In N. Schneiderman, S. M. Weiss, & P. G. Kaufmann (Eds.), *Handbook of research methods in cardiovascular behavioral medicine* (pp. 167–183). New York: Plenum.

Chapter 3

Delirium Intervention Research in Acute Care Settings

DIANE CRONIN-STUBBS
RUSH UNIVERSITY COLLEGE OF NURSING

CONTENTS

A critical appraisal of the scientific aspects of the intervention research related to the treatment and care of cognitively impaired older adults was made to assess the state of the science and to provide direction for future investigations in this understudied field. Because claims to treatment efficacy can be strengthened by attending more closely to the methodological quality of the studies, a respected model for conducting integrative research reviews (Cooper, 1989) and a priori criteria for evaluating the research literature (Cook & Campbell, 1979) were used to evaluate selected studies. As Cooper (1989) asserts, "methodological quality should be the primary criterion for decisions about how much trust to place in a study's results" (p. 64).

PROBLEM FORMULATION

Little work has been done on the care of patients with delirium in hospital settings, particularly in acute care medical and surgical settings. The dearth of intervention research in hospital settings is an important oversight because mental health problems are frequently overlooked in acute care settings (Eisdorfer, 1993). From their findings that variables associated with cognitive impairment differ in hospitalized and institutionalized elders, Roberts and Lincoln (1988) recommended setting-specific interventions. Intervention research on caring for cognitively impaired older adults in acute care medical and surgical hospital settings was the focus for the current review. Interested readers are referred to prior reviews of the literature on interventions for cognitively impaired older adults in community and home settings (Collins, Given, & Given, 1994; Given & Given, 1991; Maas & Buckwalter, 1991), long-term care settings (Maas & Buckwalter, 1991; Teitelman & Priddy, 1988); physical rehabilitation settings (Rusin, 1990); and psychiatric settings (Fopma-Loy, 1988; Raskind, Risse, & Lampe, 1987).

Older adults in all settings experience both delirium and dementia; however, "delirium is more frequently found in emergency departments and acute-care settings, and dementia in nursing homes" (Gomez & Gomez, 1989, p. 141). Delirium often accompanies serious illness in older adults; it can be life-threatening but is treatable: If interventions are timely and targeted to specific etiologies, delirium can be reversed. The focus of this review was the intervention research on caring for older adults who are cognitively impaired because of delirium.

The Research Question

The question that guided the review was, What is the state of the science of the intervention research that has been done during the past 20 years on the care and treatment of older adults with delirium in acute care medical and surgical settings?

METHODS

Available reports from nursing and interdisciplinary journals, published from 1974 to 1994, were analyzed. Integrative research review methods described by Cooper (1989) and expanded in *Meta-Analysis for Explanation: A Casebook* (Cook et al., 1992) were used. Given the small sample of reports that met inclusion criteria and the heterogeneity of interventions and outcomes represented by the reviews, a qualitative descriptive review, rather than a quantitative meta-analysis, was conducted. In a descriptive review the design features of the studies as presented by the primary researchers are objectively coded, and variations across studies are assessed. Mean effect sizes are not compared, as in a meta-analysis.

Data Collection

Because delirium and dementia are often used interchangeably in the cognitive impairment literature, the review was begun with a broad definition of cognitive impairment as related to either delirium, dementia, or pseudo-dementia. To minimize publication biases, the following diverse search methods were used: descendancy approaches (computerized searches), ancestry methods (tracing references back from current reports), and manual searches of the tables of contents of nonindexed reports. Table 3.1 summarizes the results of the literature search from these sources. A total of 332 potentially relevant reports were uncovered for review.

Data Evaluation

Results of categorizing the reports revealed that studies of interventions for cognitive impairment occurred in all settings during the study period. Most research reports were from long-term care settings ($n = 72$), acute care settings ($n = 43$), and community settings ($n = 37$), rather than psychiatric ($n = 14$) and physical rehabilitation settings ($n = 3$) (see Table 3.2). Sorting the reports by specific type of cognitive impairment revealed that delirium was studied more in acute care settings ($n = 30$; 69.8%), whereas dementia was studied

Table 3.1 Results of Literature Search from All Sources ($N = 332$)

Method	Period	Yield
Computer data bases		
PsycLIT	1/74–1/94	48
Health Plan	1/81–1/94	143
Cumulative Index to Nursing and Allied Health (CINAHL)	1/83–1/94	32
Dissertation Abstracts	1/84–1/94	19
MEDLINE	1/90–1/94	52
Manual search	6/93–1/94	20
Reports' reference lists	1/74–1/94	15
Personal solicitation	1/93–1/94	3
	TOTAL	332

Table 3.2 Number of Research Reports Representing Selected Types of Cognitive Impairment in Diverse Settings

Setting	Delirium	Dementia	Depression[a]	Total
Acute medical-surgical	30 (69.8%)	12 (27.9%)	1 (2.3%)	43
Long-term/nursing home	8 (11.1%)	61 (84.7%)	3 (4.2%)	72
Community/home	4 (10.8%)	31 (83.8%)	2 (5.4%)	37
Acute psychiatry	4 (28.6%)	10 (71.4%)	0	14
Physical rehabilitation	1 (33.3%)	1 (33.3%)	1 (33.3%)	3

[a]Reports on depression were limited to those with associated cognitive dysfunction.

more in long-term care ($n = 61$; 84.7%), community/home ($n = 31$; 83.8%), and psychiatric settings ($n = 10$; 71.4%). The difference between acute care and long-term care settings was particularly striking. If the reports actually represent the research that has occurred in the past 20 years, studies on delirium in acute care settings are more than double those on dementia. Dementia studies exceed delirium studies in long-term care settings by more than seven times. However, statements about how representative the reports are of the research that has actually occurred are made cautiously because all reviews are subject to biases. For example, no matter how thorough a reviewer is, important publications are missed, resulting in selection or sampling bias.

Using minimal criteria, the studies representing treatment of delirium in the acute care setting were selected for a critical appraisal of their scientific aspects. Those with treatment and control conditions, in which something was done for patients in a treatment group and something different was done for patients in a control group, were selected. Therefore, experimental and quasi-experimental studies of interventions for the care of acutely ill older adults (age 65 and older) were included. Nonexperimental and case studies and those with target populations averaging less than 65 years of age were excluded. Although the subset of studies representing the acute medical and surgical settings originally included 30 reports, applying the selection criteria resulted in 21 reports being dropped from the review. Nine were nonintervention studies, nine lacked control or comparison conditions, and in three reports, the average age of the samples was less than 65 years. Thus, the review was based on nine eligible studies.

Analysis and Interpretation

Using the codebook that was developed for the review, the studies' design features were analyzed and interpreted. On the basis of categories suggested by Cooper (1989), Massey and Loomis (1988), and Cook and colleagues (1992), the codebook was a 21-item, 10-page tool that included items for eliciting data about the review studies' key variables, methods, and evaluation criteria. The major categories of information that were elicited by the codebook are depicted in Table 3.3. Pretesting the codebook and assessing the interrater reliability of three randomly selected reviews resulted in changes in the ordering of the codebook items and an 86% agreement between the reviewer and an independent coder (Cohen's kappa = .72).

Scientific aspects of the studies—in particular, construct validity and statistical conclusion validity—were used to "distinguish patterns from noise" (Cook, 1993) in the studies. Construct validity refers to the congruence between theoretical and operational definitions. In the current review, construct validity was examined by coding data on the theoretical and operational definitions of the main variables, and judgments were made about their degree of correspondence.

Statistical conclusion validity refers to the power and appropriateness of the data analysis techniques used in a study (Cooper, 1989). Design features that can pose threats to the statistical conclusion validity of studies' results

Table 3.3 Major Coded Categories of Studies, Methods, Treatments, Outcomes, and Criteria for Relevance and Rigor

Studies
    Professional affiliation of author(s)
    Type of report (e.g., research, clinical, nursing, other)
    Source of report (e.g., computer database, manual search)
Methods
    Design and research question
    Theoretical and operational definitions of key variables
    Setting and sample
    Measuring mechanisms
    Data analysis
Treatment or intervention
    Content
    Implementation methods
    Implementation monitoring
Outcomes
    Description of the sample
    Main effects and significant interactions
Evaluation of relevance and rigor
    Construct validity
    External validity
    Statistical conclusion validity
    Internal validity

include the following: unreliable measures, inadequate sample sizes, inappropriate use of statistical tests, unreliable implementation of the treatment variables, and random heterogeneity in the sample of respondents, for example, data combined globally from patients younger and older than the population of interest. In the current review, random heterogeneity was controlled for by excluding studies of patients younger than 65 years. The remaining data were coded for sample size, reliability of the data collection measures, reliability of the intervention's implementation, and power and appropriateness of the statistical tests. In quantitative meta-analyses that focus on the efficacy of the outcomes, the causal relationship between the independent and dependent variables (internal validity) and the generalizability or effectiveness of the interventions in diverse settings (external validity) are additionally important.

Qualitative or descriptive analyses of the codebook data were done by conducting content analyses of the coded data to describe patterns in the review literature. With descriptive reviews, only trends are described.

RESULTS

Description of the Review Studies

The nine reports that met the study criteria had been uncovered by computerized searches and were published from 1985 to 1992 (median publication year, 1991). Seven were published articles (Cole, Fenton, Engelsmann, & Mansouri, 1991; Egbert, Parks, Short, & Burnett, 1990; Gustafson et al., 1991; Nagley, 1986; Wanich, Sullivan-Marx, Gottlieb, & Johnson, 1992; Williams, Campbell, Raynor, Mlynarczyk, & Ward, 1985; Williams-Russo, Urquhart, Sharrock, & Charlson, 1992), and two were dissertations (Miller, 1991; Sicola, 1987). Analysis of the authors' backgrounds revealed that six studies were conducted by interdisciplinary teams, done in collaboration with a member of at least one other discipline (Cole et al., 1991; Egbert et al., 1990; Gustafson et al., 1991; Wanich et al., 1992; Williams et al., 1985; Williams-Russo et al., 1992); and three were conducted by one or more nurses (Miller, 1991; Nagley, 1986; Sicola, 1987).

Analysis of setting and sample data revealed that four studies involved perioperative patients (Egbert et al., 1990; Gustafson et al., 1991; Williams et al., 1985; Williams-Russo et al., 1992), four involved medically ill patients (Miller, 1991; Nagley, 1986; Sicola, 1987; Wanich et al., 1992), and one involved both medical and postoperative surgical patients (Cole et al., 1991). Sample sizes across the nine studies ranged from 4 to 135 (median, 35) in the treatment groups and from 25 to 170 (median, 40) in the control groups. Unequal group sizes and small samples potentially weakened the power of the studies' statistical conclusions.

The average ages represented by the patients involved in the studies ranged from 67.2 years to 82.9 years (mean, 75.1 years). Gender compositions ranged from 0% to 84% female (median, 64%) and from 16% to 100% male (median, 36%). Ethnic composition of the samples was reported in only two studies (Egbert et al., 1990; Sicola, 1987), in which 80% to 90% of the respondents were Caucasian. Informed consent procedures were reported in all but two studies (Egbert et al., 1990; Gustafson et al., 1991). Given recent injunctions to include minorities and women in studies, future samples are expected to be more representative of gender and ethnicity than were the review studies.

Theoretical and Operational Definitions Used

By design, four studies were randomized clinical trials (Cole et al., 1991; Egbert et al., 1990; Sicola, 1987; Williams-Russo et al., 1992), and five were quasi-experimental. None of the studies had more than one treatment and control group. In three studies, comparisons were made from the results of previous studies, done either by the investigators (Gustafson et al., 1991; Williams et al., 1985) or by an investigator's associate (Miller, 1991). Contemporaneous comparison groups would have strengthened the validity of these studies' results.

Theoretical or conceptual frameworks were reported in only four of the nine studies, where models ($n = 3$) or a theory ($n = 1$) guided the development of the interventions tested in the studies. These included M. Powell Lawton's ecological model (Miller, 1991), Levine's Four Conservation Principles of Nursing (Nagley, 1986), Helson's Adaptation Level Theory (Sicola, 1987), and Orem's Self-Care Deficit Model (Wanich et al., 1992). Nurses were either principals or co-investigators in these four studies.

In seven studies, definitions for delirium or acute confusion ranged from informally questioning nursing personnel about the severity of patients' confusion to using criteria for delirium listed in the *Diagnostic and Statistical Manual of Mental Disorders* (DSM-III [American Psychiatric Association, 1980] or DSM-IIIR [American Psychiatric Association, 1987]). In two studies (Cole et al., 1991; Egbert et al., 1990), definitions were not given. Variability in definitions restricts comparisons among the review studies.

Also reducing the comparability of the studies was the inconsistency in what the investigators elected to use as outcomes. Although the "main goal of any intervention trial is to decrease the negative impact of the disease" (Teri et al., 1992, p. 85) and ameliorating or preventing delirium or acute confusion was the primary aim in all of the review studies, secondary outcomes were of interest in all but one study (Sicola, 1987). Most frequent were preventing iatrogenic or postoperative complications (Egbert et al., 1990; Gustafson et al., 1991; Wanich et al., 1992; Williams-Russo et al., 1992), promoting functional status or independence (Cole et al., 1991; Gustafson et al., 1991; Wanich et al., 1992; Williams-Russo et al., 1992), decreasing length of hospital stay (Gustafson et al., 1991; Wanich et al., 1992; Williams et al., 1985; Williams-Russo et al., 1992), decreasing pain (Egbert et al., 1990; Williams-Russo et al., 1992), and promoting patient satisfaction (Egbert et al., 1990; Miller, 1991) and comfort (Miller, 1991; Nagley, 1986). Despite imperatives to develop and test clinically useful interventions, only one study (Miller, 1991) specified an outcome related to the feasibility and acceptability of the intervention proto-col to the users. And although delirium can be life-threatening, only one study (Wanich et al., 1992) identified the prevention of death as an outcome secondary to decreasing incident delirium.

Although "acceptable and desirable outcomes will (and should) vary by study" (Teri et al., 1992, p. 85), not all studies a priori specified the secondary outcomes noted above, and objective methods often were not used for mea-suring them. The measurement of the primary outcome of the review studies, preventing or reducing delirium, is detailed in the following discussion.

The scientific rigor of operations for measuring delirium or acute confu-sion ranged from chart reviews and interviews to psychometrically rigorous mental status or delirium symptom checklists (see Table 3.4). Psychometrically mature tools included the Short Portable Mental Status Questionnaire (SPMSQ) (Pfeiffer, 1975) ($n = 4$), the Mini-Mental State Examination (MMSE) (Folstein, Folstein, & McHugh, 1975) ($n = 2$), the Crichton Geriatric Behavioral Rating Scale (CGBRS) (Robinson, 1961) ($n = 1$), and the NEECHAM Confusion Scale (Neelon, Champagne, McConnell, Carlson, & Funk, 1992) ($n = 1$). The SPMSQ and the MMSE are cognitive status tests, and the CGBRS measures functional disability, abnormal behavior, orientation, and comprehension. Only the NEECHAM Scale specifically measures delirium.

Immature tools included investigator-developed tools for delirium or con-fusion assessment ($n = 6$) and checklists or questionnaires derived from DSM III (1980) or DSM IIIR (1978, 1987) criteria ($n = 2$). Equal numbers of mature ($n = 8$) and immature tools ($n = 8$) were used across the studies. However, six of these were cognitive status tests (SPMSQ, MMSE); only one mature tool (NEECHAM) was specific to delirium. This may reflect the developmental stages of cognitive status and delirium research, respectively.

None of the studies that used either the SPMSQ or the MMSE also used an adjunctive psychometrically mature tool to specifically measure delirium. In one study, the SPMSQ was used alone (Egbert et al., 1990). In two others, it was used with immature, investigator-developed confusion-assessment tools (Nagley, 1986; Williams et al., 1985). In the study by Cole and colleagues (1991), the SPMSQ was included in a battery of tools that assessed related but divergent conditions (e.g., anxiety, depression, abnormal behaviors, and func-

Table 3.4 Data Collection Methods in the Review Studies ($N = 9$) for Measuring Delirium or Acute Confusional State or Acute Confustion

	Mental Status Tools		Delirium (ACS) Tools		Clinical Methods		
	SPMSQ	MMSE	Mature	Immature[a]	Onservation	Records	Interviews
Cole et al., 1991	x		x	x	x	x	x
Egbert et al., 1990	x						
Gustafson et al., 1991				x		x	
Miller, 1991	x		x	x	x		x
Nagley, 1986	x			x			
Sicola, 1987		x		x			
Wanich et al., 1992		x		x	x	x	x
Williams et al., 1985	x			x	x	x	x
Williams-Russo et al., 1992				x	x	x	x

[a]Immature tools include clinical assessment tools (e.g., tools incorporating DSM-III or DSM-IIIR criteria) and investigator-developed tools without apparent psychometric information.

tional disability). Delirium was not measured by psychometrically mature methods in the review studies.

By virtue of its multidimensionality and its overlap with other types of cognitive impairment (e.g., dementia and pseudodementia), the measurement of delirium optimally involves multiple and diverse methods to contribute to the validity and adequacy of construct representation. However, in only one-third of the studies were more than two methods to measure delirium used (Miller, 1991; Wanich et al., 1992; Williams et al., 1985). Also, independent, double-blinded raters and direct observations of studies' outcome variables ideally are used to corroborate paper-and-pencil measures. Although observational methods were used for this purpose in Miller's (1991) study, none of the studies consistently used raters who were blind to the purposes of the studies and to membership in the treatment and control groups.

Diverse definitions across the studies, the inadequacy of construct and operational representation of delirium within the studies, and the inadequate correspondence between theoretical and operational definitions suggest that the review studies generally lacked concept-to-operations congruence or construct validity. Systematic bias, introduced by nonstandardized and non-objective data collection methods, threatens the statistical conclusion validity of the studies' results. Without construct validity and statistical conclusion validity, the construct validity of the interventions and their efficacy also may be threatened.

Examining the reliability of the studies' measures, psychometric information for the tools either were not reported (Egbert et al., 1990; Gustafson et al., 1991; Williams-Russo et al., 1992) or psychometric information was reported from previous studies (Wanich et al., 1992; Williams et al., 1985). In only two studies were more than one form of reliability and validity reported (Miller, 1991; Sicola, 1987). Only three of the five studies that used investigator-developed assessment tools reported psychometric information about the new tools (Miller, 1991; Nagley, 1986; Sicola, 1987). In general, psychometric information was either lacking or minimal.

Across the nine studies, the most common data analysis procedures were analysis of variance (ANOVA; one-way, factorial, repeated measures [$n = 5$]), t-tests ($n = 5$), multiple logistic regression ($n = 4$), chi square ($n = 4$), and nonparametric ANOVA ($n = 2$). Although the choice of parametric and nonparametric procedures was appropriate for the studies' sample sizes, consistent use of power analyses, which were reported in only three studies (Cole et al., 1991; Egbert et al., 1990; Williams-Russo et al., 1992), would have promoted confidence in the studies' statistical conclusions.

The reliability of the implementation of the treatment variables also contributes to the statistical conclusion validity of the studies' results. The interventions tested in the review studies and the methods used for assessing and monitoring the implementation of the interventions are described in the following section.

Interventions Tested

The range of interventions that were tested in the review studies included a geriatric psychiatry consultation service (Cole et al., 1991); methods of administering postoperative pain medication (Egbert et al., 1990; Williams-Russo et al., 1992); perioperative management of physiological parameters, including treatment of postoperative complications (Gustafson et al., 1991); and environmental management of, for example, excessive or "meaningless" stimuli (Miller, 1991; Sicola, 1987; Williams et al., 1985). Five of the nine studies evaluated intervention programs that combined reorientation activities and sensory deficit management with "good patient care" interventions, such as managing pain (Sicola, 1987), monitoring medications (Wanich et al. 1992), promoting urinary elimination (Sicola, 1987; Williams et al., 1985) and mobility (Nagley, 1986; Sicola, 1987; Wanich et al., 1992; Williams et al., 1985), maximizing independence in activities of daily living (Miller, 1991), and responding to patients' needs for financial assistance and housing (Sicola, 1987). Most review studies, then, tested multifaceted combinations of interventions.

These multifaceted interventions are laudable from comprehensive patient care perspectives. However, scientifically, it is difficult to identify causal agents or active ingredients in the intervention packages. Controlled conditions and large sample sizes are required to determine the contributions of individual and potentially interacting treatment components to the studies' outcomes. The small samples and the complex, potentially overlapping, nonindependent interventions may explain the nonsignificant findings in seven of the nine review studies. Statistical power may have been weakened, and type II errors may have occurred. As a result, significant active ingredients may have been masked.

Another important contributor to type II error and a main threat to statistical conclusion validity is unreliable implementation of the interventions or treatments, which can affect the maximum potential effect of interventions and distort conclusions made about the power of their efficacy. Three of the nine studies lacked provision for implementation assessment and monitoring (Cole et al., 1991; Sicola, 1987; Wanich et al., 1992). Direct or indirect physiological methods were used in the perioperative studies to assess implementation; they included monitoring of amounts of analgesia used (Williams-Russo et al., 1992), serum morphine levels (Egbert et al., 1990), and arterial blood gases (Gustafson et al., 1991). The nursing care studies typically validated interventions through self-report and observational methods, such as flow sheets that were completed either by the nurses implementing the interventions (Miller, 1991; Nagley, 1986; Williams et al., 1985) or by nonblinded observers (Miller, 1991). For optimal objectivity, assessment of the interventions' implementation should be done by trained and blinded research staff who are not involved in treatment implementation or the care of the patients. In addition, indirect measures of treatment implementation may encompass other variables than those under study. Unvalidated self-report data are typically replete with social desirability bias. Direct observations by independent, double-blinded evaluators and ongoing, intermittently scheduled monitoring with psychometrically rigorous measures promotes confidence in the implementation of treatment variables.

DISCUSSION

Of the 332 reports representing the past generation of studies of cognitively impaired older adults, only 30 (9%) represented research-based care of patients with delirium in acute care settings. This may reflect the underrecognition of delirium in medical and surgical patients described by Gutmann (1988) and Lipowski (1989). However, it is possible that reports were missed in searching the literature due to unintended selection biases.

Nine of the 30 reports that were uncovered met the inclusion criterion of using comparison or control groups in their evaluation of treatment efficacy. Although the search covered the past 20 years, no studies were found prior to 1985 that met this criterion. Although studies prior to 1985 may have used other terms for delirium or acute confusion (e.g., postcardiotomy psychosis) and would not have been uncovered in the search, those that were uncovered could be characterized as preexperimental.

No scientifically robust or consistently rigorous studies for responding to the delirium of the hospitalized older adult were found in this appraisal. This state of the science may be related to the threats to construct and statistical conclusion validity that were identified rather than to the inadequacy of the interventions that were tested. Many studies lacked samples large enough to draw powerful conclusions. Both large- and small-sample studies had problems with unreliable measures of primary and secondary outcomes. Most problematic to construct validity was inadequate representation of the delirium construct that the measures were intended to operationalize. Statistical conclusion validity was problematic because of the lack of reliable methods for implementing and monitoring the interventions under study. This may reflect the lack of psychometrically rigorous tools for both measuring delirium and assessing the implementation of the interventions.

Research in this area, then, seems to be vulnerable to the threats to validity that plague most field studies. In their review of dementia care research, Teri et al. (1992) summarized the following "overriding concerns" (p. 85) that existed in that body of intervention research: the need for specific theoretical and operational definitions of targeted symptoms or diseases; the use of mature, psychometrically established and clinically valid measures; the use of specific, objective criteria for evaluating change in outcomes that can be ascribed to treatment conditions; and the use of comprehensive and diverse methods of assessing both treatments and outcomes. The current review studies were vulnerable to validity threats related to adequacy of construct representation, unreliable measures, inadequate power, and unreliable treatment implementation, assessment, and monitoring. The recent development of symptom checklists to supplement mental status tests for detecting and differentiating delirium from other forms of cognitive impairment may assist future researchers in correcting some of the problems identified in the past generation of acute care studies. As suggested by Teri et al., to determine if an intervention trial decreases the negative impact of symptoms or diseases, "both focused indices of change and comprehensive assessment strategies are needed" (p. 85).

Conclusions about the field of delirium intervention research are tempered by threats to the validity of the findings of this review. Because the review reports were restricted to those that met the inclusion criterion of including control or comparison groups, the review was limited to experimental and quasi-experimental studies. Nine of 30 potential reports met the inclusion criteria. The small sample of reports cannot be assumed to represent the field of delirium intervention research. By using restrictive inclusion criteria, thereby choosing potential methodological quality over representativeness, "selectivity limits the generalizability of conclusions drawn" (Bryant & Wortman, 1984, p. 9) to those studies with characteristics that are similar to the nine studies in the review. However, general recommendations about the future direction of delirium intervention research can be advanced from the patterns that were identified across the review studies.

DIRECTIONS FOR THE FUTURE

The research to date supports the prevalence of delirium during and following inpatient stays; however, the field of caring for hospitalized older adults with delirium seems to be in the early phases of development. Research-based protocols require further testing in randomized clinical trials or meticulously designed quasi-experimental studies before they are ready for translation to the care of cognitively impaired older adults. Before probing causal inferences about the direct effects of the treatment variables on both primary and secondary outcomes (internal validity) and before attempting to generalize findings of intervention studies to diverse populations, settings, and time periods (external validity), it is necessary to give more attention to strengthening construct validity and statistical conclusion validity in the design of future studies. According to Cook and Campbell (1979), a priori attention to construct validity contributes to external validity; a priori attention to statistical conclusion validity fosters internal validity.

Evaluating the efficacy and, eventually, the effectiveness of targeted interventions requires further research. More studies also are needed on evaluating the validity and reliability of intervention programs, including implementation assessment and monitoring, and on promoting the use of intervention protocols in patient care settings.

Consistent with the review of the dementia care research (Teri et al., 1992), studies of caring for patients with delirium need to "integrate biomedical and behavioral expertise to develop methodologically rigorous study designs where theoretically sound, clinically judicious, and scientifically rigorous research protocols" (p. 86) are designed and tested. From the findings of the current review, clarification of what comprises delirium (construct validity) and selection of appropriate outcome measures (statistical conclusion validity) will guide the development and evaluation of valid treatment packages. Most essential outcomes include the reversal of delirium, which is a treatable form of cognitive impairment, and the prevention of death.

In the interim, patients are discharged from the hospital with impaired cognition that potentially could be reversed. Although family members and patients, as well as professional caregivers, may assume that impairments in mental status naturally coexist with increasing age or medical illness, research designed to develop and test interventions aimed at identifying, preventing, and treating the diverse and complex causes of delirium will contribute to nursing care with improved outcomes for our medically and mentally ill older adults.

ACKNOWLEDGMENTS

This review was funded in part by the National Institute of Mental Health, National Institutes of Health (Grant No. 5 K07 MH00953-03). The author gratefully acknowledges Thomas D. Cook, PhD, Northwestern University, for enlightenment and direction; Frederick J. Kviz, PhD, University of Illinois at Chicago, for scientific and editorial input; Lois B. Taft, DNSc, RN, Rush University, for critical appraisal of earlier drafts of the manuscript; and Maura

Capaul, Rush University, and Rebecca S. Woodham, University of Iowa, for participation in interrater reliability assessments and preparation of the final manuscript.

REFERENCES

American Psychiatric Association. (1978). *Diagnostic and statistical manual of mental disorders*, (3rd ed.). Washington, DC: Task Force on Nomenclature and Statistics.

American Psychiatric Association. (1980). *Diagnostic and statistical manual of mental disorders* (3rd ed.). Washington, DC: American Psychiatric Press.

American Psychiatric Association. (1987). *Diagnostic and statistical manual of mental disorders* (3rd ed., rev.). Washington, DC: Author.

Bryant, F., & Wortman, P. M. (1984). Methodological issues in meta-analysis of quasi-experiments. In W. H. Yeaton & P. M. Wortman (Eds.), *Issues in data synthesis: New directions in program evaluation* (pp. 5–24). San Francisco: Jossey-Bass.

Cole, M. G., Fenton, F. R., Engelsmann, G., & Mansouri, I. (1991). Effectiveness of geriatric psychiatry consultation in an acute care hospital: A randomized clinical trial. *Journal of the American Geriatrics Society, 39*, 1183–1188.

Collins, C. E., Given, B. A., & Given, C. W. (1994). Interventions with family caregivers of persons with Alzheimer's disease. *Nursing Clinics of North America, 29*, 195–207.

Cook, T. D., & Campbell, D. T. (1979). *Quasi-experimentation: Design and analysis issues for field settings*. Boston: Houghton Mifflin.

Cook, T. D., Cooper, H., Cordray, D. S., Hartmann, H., Hedges, L. V., Light, R. J., Louis, T. A., & Mosteller, F. (1992). *Meta-analysis for explanation: A casebook*. New York: Russell Sage Foundation.

Cook, T. (1993). *Designs for descriptive causal research in field settings, Part II*. Northwestern University, Evanston, IL: Postdoctoral Research Seminar.

Cooper, H. M. (1989). *Integrating research: A guide for literature reviews* (2nd ed.). In L. Bickman & D. J. Rog (Eds.), *Applied social research methods series* (Vol. 2). Newbury Park, CA: Sage Publications.

Egbert, A. M., Parks, L. H., Short, L. M., & Burnett, M. L. (1990). Randomized trial of postoperative patient-controlled analgesia vs intramuscular narcotics in frail elderly men. *Archives of Internal Medicine, 150*, 1897–1903.

Eisdorfer, C. (1993). Three overviews of mental health and aging. *Gerontologist, 33*, 570–571.

Folstein, M. F., Folstein, S., & McHugh, P. R. (1975). Mini-Mental State: A practical method for grading the cognitive state of patients for the clinician. *Journal of Psychiatric Research, 12*, 189–198.

Fopma-Loy, J. (1988). Wandering: Causes, consequences, and care. *Journal of Psychosocial Nursing and Mental Health Services, 26*(5), 8–18.

Given, B. A., & Given, C. W. (1991). Family caregiving for the elderly. In J. J. Fitzpatrick & J. S. Stevenson (Eds.), *Annual review of nursing research* (Vol. 9, pp. 77–101). New York: Springer Publishing Co.

Gomez, G., & Gomez, E. A. (1989). Dementia? Or delirium?: Here's help in sorting it out. *Geriatric Nursing: American Journal of Care for the Aging, 10,* 141–142.

Gustafson, Y., Brannstrom, B., Berggren, D., Ragnarsson, J. I., Sigaard, J., Bucht, G., Reiz, S., Norberg, A., & Winblad, B. (1991). A geriatric-anesthesiologic program to reduce acute confusional states in elderly patients treated for femoral neck fractures. *Journal of the American Geriatrics Society, 39,* 655–662.

Gutmann, D. (1988). Late onset pathogenesis: Dynamic models. *Topics in Geriatric Rehabilitation, 3*(4), 1–8.

Lipowski, Z. J. (1989). Delirium in the elderly patient. *New England Journal of Medicine, 320,* 578–582.

Maas, M. L., & Buckwalter, K. C. (1991). Alzheimer's disease. In J. J. Fitzpatrick & J. S. Stevenson (Eds.), *Annual review of nursing research* (Vol. 9, pp. 19–55). New York: Springer Publishing Co.

Massey, J., & Loomis, M. (1988). When should nurses use research findings? *Applied Nursing Research, 1,* 32–40.

Miller, J. D. (1991). A clinical study to pilot test the environmental optimization interventions protocol. *Dissertations Abstracts International, 53*(02) 772B.

Nagley, S. J. (1986). Predicting and preventing confusion in your patients. *Journal of Gerontological Nursing, 12*(3), 27–31.

Neelon, V. J., Champagne, M. T., McConnell, E., Carlson, J., & Funk, S. (1992). Use of the NEECHAM Confusion Scale to assess acute confusional states of hospitalized older patients. In S. G. Funk, E. M. Tornquist, M. T. Champagne, & R. A. Wiese (Eds.), *Key aspects of elder care: Managing falls, incontinence, and cognitive impairment* (pp. 278–289). New York: Springer Publishing Co.

Pfeiffer, E. (1975). A Short Portable Mental Status Questionnaire for the assessment of organic brain deficit in elderly patients. *Journal of the American Geriatrics Society, 23,* 433–441.

Raskind, M. A., Risse, S. C., & Lampe, T. H. (1987). Dementia and antipsychotic drugs. *Journal of Clinical Psychiatry, 48*(Suppl.), 16–18.

Roberts, B. L., & Lincoln, R. E. (1988). Cognitive disturbance in hospitalized and institutionalized elders. *Research in Nursing and Health, 11,* 309–319.

Robinson, R. (1961). Some problems of clinical trials in elderly people. *Gerontology Clinician, 3,* 247–257.

Rusin, M. J. (1990). Stroke rehabilitation: A geropsychological perspective. *Archives of Physical Medicine and Rehabilitation, 71,* 914–922.

Sicola, V. R. (1987). Daily orientation program's effect on hospitalized elderly medical patients predicted to be at risk for an acute confusional state. *Dissertation Abstracts International, 48*(04), 1008, AAC 8715015.

Teitelman, J. L., & Priddy, M. J. (1988). From psychological theory to practice: Improving frail elders' quality of life through control-enhancing interventions. *Journal of Applied Gerontology, 7,* 298–315.

Teri, L., Rabins, P., Whitehouse, P., Berg, L., Risberg, B., Sunderland, T., Eichelman, B., & Creighton, P. (1992). Management of behavior disturbance in Alzheimer disease: Current knowledge and future directions. *Alzheimer Disease and Associated Disorders, 6*(2), 77–88.

Wanich, C. K., Sullivan-Marx, E. M., Gottlieb, G. L., & Johnson, J. C. (1992). Functional status outcomes of a nursing intervention in hospitalized elderly. *Image: Journal of Nursing Scholarship, 24,* 201–207.

Williams, M. A., Campbell, E. B., Raynor, W. J., Mlynarczyk, S. M., & Ward, S. E. (1985). Reducing acute confusional states in elderly patients with hip fractures. *Research in Nursing and Health, 8*, 329–337.

Williams-Russo, P., Urquhart, B. L., Sharrock, N. E., & Charlson, M. E. (1992). Postoperative delirium: Predictors and prognosis in elderly orthopedic patients. *Journal of the American Geriatrics Society, 40*, 759–767.

Chapter 4

Smoking Cessation Interventions in Chronic Illness

MARY ELLEN WEWERS
COLLEGE OF NURSING
THE OHIO STATE UNIVERSITY

KAREN L. AHIJEVYCH
COLLEGE OF NURSING
THE OHIO STATE UNIVERSITY

CONTENTS

The health consequences of tobacco abuse are well documented; cigarette smoking is a major risk factor for both coronary artery disease and chronic obstructive pulmonary disease and represents the major cause of cancer deaths in the United States (U.S. Department of Health and Human Services, 1989). Tobacco use has been described as the single most preventable cause of premature morbidity and mortality. Although the majority of tobacco cessation research has been focused on prevention and cessation among smokers prior to disease, clinicians and researchers have begun to recognize that cessation interventions with ill populations of smokers have merit (Emmons & Goldstein, 1992). Among smokers with various comorbid conditions, the benefits of cessation include, to name a few, a reduced risk for (a) recurrence of acute myocardial infarction (U.S. Department of Health and Human Services, 1990a), (b) incidence of a second primary malignant tumor after diagnosis with small cell lung cancer (Richardson et al., 1993), (c) decline in pulmonary function among emphysematous patients (U.S. Department of Health and Human Services, 1990a), (d) macroproteinuria and proliferative neuropathy in noninsulin dependent diabetics (Mulhauser, Sawicki, & Berger, 1986), (e) lower extremity ischemia or amputation in persons with peripheral vascular disease (Bloom, Stevick, & Lemmon, 1990), and (f) relapse among recovering alcoholics (DeSoto, O'Donnell, & DeSoto, 1989). Finally, because smoking has been shown to complicate illnesses and conditions that are more prevalent in the elderly, cessation benefits have been reported to continue with aging (Achkar, 1985; Mellstrom, Rundgren, Jagenburg, Steen, & Svanborg, 1982; Somerville, Faulkner, & Langham, 1986).

Forty-six million Americans are cigarette smokers (Centers for Disease Control, 1991). Current projections for the year 2000 suggest that 22% of the adult population will be smokers and that 30% of adults with a high school education or less will smoke (Pierce, Fiore, Novotny, Hatziandreu, & Davis, 1989). Although previous cessation approaches have been successfully implemented for the most part, with well-educated healthy populations of smokers, future programs must continue to develop innovative strategies to effectively reach more smokers. As such, recent cessation efforts have involved delivery of an intervention in inpatient or outpatient health settings where a smoker is being treated for a concomitant comorbid condition.

This chapter is focused on a review of cessation intervention research among smokers with chronic comorbid conditions (i.e., in the presence of illness) in inpatient or outpatient settings. The critical review includes a synthesis of the research findings, with specific attention to variables that have been addressed, and directions for future research investigations. The review consists of published, peer-reviewed reports of randomized and other controlled clinical trials of smoking cessation, from 1975 to the present, among smokers with comorbid conditions, that included an outcome measure of smoking status at a minimum of 6 months postintervention. Among cessation experts, follow-up outcome evaluation of abstinence at 6 and/or 12 months is considered valid for measuring success (Schwartz, 1987). Twenty-three studies met these criteria.

SMOKING BEHAVIOR

Theoretical Foundations

Tobacco use, which occurs primarily through smoking, is a behavior influenced by pharmacological, psychological, social, and environmental factors (Fisher, Haire-Joshu, Morgan, Rehberg, & Rost, 1990). Nicotine, the major addictive agent in tobacco, provides both euphoriant and sedating effects and serves as powerful pharmacological reinforcement for maintenance of the behavior (U.S. Department of Health and Human Services, 1988). In addition to its pharmacological characteristics, smoking involves a strong psychological dependence in that smokers report engaging in the behavior to alleviate negative affective symptoms, such as tension, anxiety, boredom, and irritability (Shiffman, 1979). The subsequent reduction of dysphoric states leads, in turn, to continued pursuit of the behavior. Social and environmental motives also influence the behavior. The majority of smokers are surrounded by family members and friends who engage in the behavior, providing strong cues to continue smoking (McIntyre-Kingsolver, Lichtenstein, & Mermelstein, 1983; Ockene, Benfari, Nuttall, Hurwitz, & Ockene, 1982).

A model developed by Prochaska and DiClemente (1983) categorizes persons along a continuum of behavioral change. According to the model, as applied to smoking behavior, persons may be classified into different stages of cessation, which range from precontemplation, or not thinking about cessation, to maintenance, that is, abstinence from smoking for a specified period of time. Other stages of this continuum include contemplation, preparation, and action. According to Prochaska (1992), only 10% to 20% of smokers are in the preparation phase, and 30% to 40% can be considered contemplators. Thus, the remaining group of smokers (40% to 60%) are in the precontemplation stage of behavior change.

To address the multivariate nature of the behavior, cessation interventions have generally included multicomponent treatment programs that include: (a) behavioral modification therapy aimed at substituting other behaviors for smoking, (b) health education counseling, and (c) pharmacotherapy, primarily in the form of nicotine replacement. In addition, based on Prochaska's behavior change model, different approaches to cessation are recommended for each stage of cessation. These approaches, labeled "processes of change," are stage-specific and may vary, depending on the smoker's stage of cessation (e.g., precontemplation vs. action).

Outcome Measures

Five to six serious quit attempts are required before a smoker achieves permanent cessation (Fisher et al., 1990). National annual cessation, or quit, rates are 0.5% among adult cigarette smokers aged 20 and older (U.S. Department of Health and Human Services, 1990b). The effectiveness of cessation interventions has been evaluated in the past by a variety of measures ranging from self- and collaborator reports of current smoking to biochemical verification of abstinence. Abstinence is categorized as (a) point prevalence—abstinent at a particular time, (b) continuous—abstinent since the occurrence of cessation attempt, or (c) prolonged—abstinent for a specified period, such as 6 or 12 months (Velicer, Prochaska, Rossi, & Snow, 1992). A phenomenon known as the "bogus" pipeline procedure is often used to enhance the accuracy of smoking self-report (Velicer et al., 1992). The procedure, which involves obtaining a biological sample in concert with self-report of smoking behavior, often increases accuracy of reporting because the person assumes the sample can be analyzed to confirm smoking status. Point prevalence abstinence outcomes are reported in this review. To evaluate the intervention's effectiveness more accurately, all abstinence rates were adjusted to reflect sample size at entry into the study and may differ from rates reported by the actual investigators.

The accuracy of self-report has been questioned (Velicer et al., 1992), especially among populations of smokers in which there there is a "high demand" (i.e., need to report abstinence) for nonsmoking, as is often the case with smokers who have a diagnosis that is tobacco-related, such as coronary artery disease. For this subset of smokers, it has been recommended that abstinence be confirmed biochemically. Cotinine, the primary metabolite of nicotine, is considered the most valid marker of tobacco smoke exposure (Benowitz, 1983). Cotinine is specific for nicotine, has concentrations 10 times greater than that of nicotine, remains fairly constant, and detects light and intermittent smoking (Benowitz, 1983). Cotinine levels in plasma, saliva, and urine are highly correlated (Jarvis, Tunstall-Pedoe, Feyerabend, Vesey, & Saloojee, 1984). Cotinine is a good indicator of tobacco exposure because it has a relatively long half-life of 16 to 20 hours (Benowitz, Kuyt, Jacob, Jones, & Osman, 1983). However, cotinine is not an appropriate biomarker for participants who are being treated with nicotine replacement because cotinine will be detected among abstinent persons on nicotine pharmacotherapy. In these studies, expired air carbon monoxide (ECO_a), a by-product of cigarette smoke with a half-life of 4 to 6 hours, is often substituted as a biochemical outcome measure. Some earlier studies used thiocyanate, a metabolite of hydrogen cyanide that is present in tobacco, as a biomarker of tobacco exposure (Benowitz, 1983). Because thiocyanate levels are often increased among persons who consume certain types of vegetables, the specificity of the measure is diminished, thus reducing its suitability in smoking cessation research.

RESEARCH FINDINGS

Comorbid Conditions

The majority of cessation intervention studies have included smokers with a cardiovascular diagnosis of acute myocardial infarction or coronary artery disease. Four inpatient treatment approaches involved multicomponent programs of health education counseling and behavioral modification techniques (DeBusk et al., 1994; Ockene et al., 1992; Rigotti, McKool, & Shiffman, 1994; Taylor, Houston-Miller, Haskell, & DeBusk, 1988). Of these, three programs were delivered by a nurse and one by a health educator; all providers were trained in smoking cessation therapy, and all programs included telephone follow-up, ranging from one time to monthly calls during the first 6 months posttreatment. In these studies, researchers examined the effectiveness of intervening during hospitalization during the postinfarction or pre– and postcoronary artery bypass surgery recovery phases, and all involved biochemical confirmation of quit rates at 6 or 12 months postintervention.

Two studies, instituted during outpatient cardiac rehabilitation treatment, examined the effects of long-term exercise programs (12 to 23 weeks), in combination with printed cessation materials and counseling on abstinence from smoking (Sivarajan, Newton, Almes, Kempf, & Bruce, 1983; Taylor et al., 1988). One of these studies involved biochemical confirmation (Taylor et al., 1988), whereas the earlier investigation (Sivarajan et al., 1983) relied solely on self-report of abstinence.

Four studies were conducted among pulmonary patients with a diagnosis of emphysema or chronic bronchitis (Anthonisen et al., 1994; Pederson, Lefcoe, & Wood, 1983; Pederson, Wanklin, & Lefcoe, 1991; Tønnesen et al., 1988). Two of these investigations were begun during hospitalization, and involved printed cessation materials (Pederson et al., 1983, 1991). In one of these reports, advice to quit was delivered by a nonhealth care provider who was specifically trained to deliver smoking cessation information. Neither of these studies included any outpatient follow-up. Two studies examined the effect of nicotine replacement (gum) and behavior modification counseling on cessation and were performed in an outpatient clinic environment over 10 weeks (Anthonisen et al., 1994) and 16 weeks (Tønnesen et al., 1988). The Lung Health Study (LHS) (Anthonisen et al., 1994) included extended follow-up treatment aimed at relapse prevention. Three of the four studies cited above included biochemical confirmation of abstinence at 6 or 12 months postintervention. The Lung Health Study followed participants for up to 5 years and described continuous abstinence, as well as point prevalence quit rates.

Three studies included smokers with cardiovascular or pulmonary conditions (British Thoracic Society, 1983; Hall, Bachman, Henderson, Barstow, & Jones, 1983; Prue, Davis, Martin, & Moss, 1983). Interventions were conducted in outpatient settings, except for 20% of subjects who were inpatients in the British Thoracic study (1983). Intensity of the intervention varied from brief face-to-face advice (British Thoracic Society, 1983) to telephone contact every 2 weeks (Prue et al., 1983) to six 90-minute sessions over 3 weeks with 60-minute booster sessions at weeks 5 and 8 (Hall et al., 1983). The British Thoracic Society study (1983) extended data collection points to 1, 3, 6, and

12 months postintervention. Outcome measures of the studies were obtained at 6 months by corroboration (Prue et al., 1983) or by ECO_a (Hall et al., 1983) and at 12 months with carboxyhemoglobin and thiocyanate (British Thoracic Society, 1983).

Inpatient smokers with various diagnoses were the focus of two studies (Stevens, Glasgow, Hollis, Lichtenstein, & Vogt, 1993; Campbell, Prescott, & Tjeder-Burton, 1991). Brief face-to-face advice and support and nicotine gum or placebo were used in the Campbell et al. study (1991); a 20-minute bedside counseling session, a 12-minute videotape tailored to inpatients, follow-up phone calls, and bimonthly newsletters were included in the Stevens et al. (1993) study. Outcome was assessed by self-report at 3 and 12 months (Stevens et al., 1993) and via ECO_a at 12 months by Campbell et al. (1991).

Recently, three cessation intervention studies in samples with a specific diagnosis were reported: peripheral vascular disease (Power, Brown, & Makin, 1992), diabetes mellitus (Sawicki, Didjurgeit, Muhlhauser, & Berger, 1993), and head and neck cancer (Gritz et al., 1993). Participants were identified in clinic settings. Intervention intensity ranged from 1 45-minute counseling session (Power et al., 1992) to advice plus 6 booster sessions (Gritz et al., 1993) to 10 90-minute sessions with multicomponent aspects (Sawicki et al., 1993). Outcomes were measured with cotinine at 6 months in all three, with an additional 12-month data collection in the head and neck cancer sample.

Elderly persons were the focus of two interventions (Rimer et al., 1994; Vetter & Ford, 1990). Both samples were recruited by mail, either from clients of a large family practice clinic (Vetter & Ford, 1990) or from the readership of *Modern Maturity* (Rimer et al., 1994). Face-to-face physician advice with nurse follow-up over 6 months was implemented in the family practice setting; two forms of a mailed intervention and two phone calls were aspects of the research with a national sample (Rimer et al., 1994). Vetter and Ford (1990) used ECO_a to confirm outcome biochemically at 6 months, and Rimer et al. (1994) collected self-reported smoking status information at 12 months.

Three investigations implemented cessation intervention with patients in treatment for substance abuse (Burling, Marshall, & Seidner, 1991; Hurt et al., 1994; Story & Stark, 1991). Methadone maintenance clinic participants were the sample in one study (Story & Stark, 1991); in others the intervention was implemented with inpatients in treatment for alcohol or other drug dependencies. Burling et al. (1991) conducted outcome measures at 6 months, whereas others assessed effect at 12 months.

Quit rates in experimental groups of the 23 studies reviewed ranged from 0% to 71%; control group quit rates ranged from 0% to 74% (Table 4.1). Three studies were associated with no differences between experimental and control group abstinence rates (Burling et al., 1991; Campbell et al., 1991; Rigotti et al., 1994). In five studies, control group abstinence rates averaged 8% greater, as compared to experimental group rates (Gritz et al., 1993; Pederson et al., 1983; Sawicki et al., 1993; Story & Stark, 1991; Taylor et al., 1988). Finally, for 11 studies, the experimental abstinence rates were, on average, 14.8% greater, when contrasted to control group rates (Anthonisen et al., 1994; DeBusk et al., 1994; Hurt et al., 1994; Ockene et al., 1992; Pederson et al., 1991; Power et al., 1992; Prue et al., 1983; Stevens et al., 1993; Taylor et al., 1990). Four studies were associated with multiple interventions and did not contain a "true" control group (British Thoracic Society, 1983; Hall et al., 1983; Rimer et al., 1994; Sivarajan et al., 1983).

Pertinent Variables

Sociodemographic Factors.   Mean age of subjects enrolled in the studies ranged from 36 to greater than 60. The majority of subjects were fairly well educated. Mean educational level was generally at 12 years, and many studies included smokers who had at least some college education. The overwhelming majority of subjects were male, and all investigations were conducted among Caucasian smokers with the exception of two studies that included 3% (Anthonisen et al., 1994) and 36% non-White subjects (Burling et al., 1991). In studies where marital status was described, about one-half of participants were currently married. However, for the most part, smoking behavior of significant others was not described. Dependence on other drugs was addressed only in those three studies of patients in drug treatment programs (Burling et al., 1991; Hurt et al., 1994; Story & Stark, 1991). Three investigations specifically excluded persons who were alcohol abusers, and 17 reports did not describe alcohol or drug use patterns of participants.

Stages of Smoking Cessation.   Three studies described subjects' stage of smoking cessation with sample characteristics. Two reports specifically categorized subjects, according to stage at baseline (Gritz et al., 1993; Ockene et al., 1992), and one study inferred that those subjects who had made a serious attempt to quit in the past year were in the preparation stage of cessation (Rimer et al., 1994).

Type of Treatment.   Counseling ranging from a few minutes to a 45-minute session was the primary intervention in seven studies (British Thoracic Society, 1983; Campbell et al., 1991; Gritz et al., 1993; Power et al., 1992; Sawicki et al., 1993; Stevens et al., 1993; Vetter & Ford, 1990). Two of these also offered nicotine replacement in the form of gum, two added printed materials, and one sent reminder postcards. Although one-time advice sometimes yields lower quit rates than more intensive treatment, the potential for reaching many smokers may offset this limitation.

Table 4.1 Abstinence Rates (%) at 6 and/or 12 Months, Significance, and Sample Size of Reviewed Studies by Comorbid Condition

Author, Date	Experimental, 6 Months	Control, 6 Months	Experimental, 12 Months	Control, 12 Months	Sample Size (N)
Cardiovascular					
DeBusk et al., 1994	68.7	55.4 Significance not reported	70	53 p = .03	585
Ockene et al., 1992	45.1	34.4 p = .06	33	23 p = .07	267
Rigotti et al., 1994			51	51 NS	87
Sivarajan et al., 1983[a]	33.3 44.2	37.8 NS			119
Taylor et al., 1988	31	39 NS			68
Taylor et al., 1990			60.7	31.7 p = .001	173
Pulmonary					
Anthonisen et al., 1994	35	10 Significance not reported			5887
Pederson et al., 1983	14.3	25 NS			75

Pederson et al., 1991	28.6	19.4 NS			74
Tønnesen et al., 1988			33.3	3.7 $p < .001$	173
Cardiopulmonary					
British Thoracic Society 1983[a]			11.1 10.9 13.9 10.0	NS	1550
Hall et al., 1983[a]	26.3 6.3	NS			35
Prue et al., 1983	26.7	10 Significance not reported			40
Inpatients					
Campbell et al., 1991	19.6	20 NS			212
Stevens et al., 1993			21	16.7 $p = .068$	1119
Specific diagnosis					
Gritz et al., 1993	71.4	73.9 NS			186

(continued)

Table 4.1 (*Continued*)

Author, Date	Experimental, 6 Months	Control, 6 Months	Experimental, 12 Months	Control, 12 Months	Sample Size (N)
Power et al., 1992	27.5	20 Significance not reported			60
Sawicki et al., 1993	5	16 NS			89
Substance abuse patients					
Burling et al., 1991	0	0 Significance not reported			39
Hurt et al., 1994			11.8	0 p = .027	101
Story & Stark, 1991	0	9 Significance not reported			22
Elderly					
Rimer et al., 1994[a]			20 19	15 p = .01	1867
Vetter & Ford, 1990	14.3	8.5 p < .05			471

[a]Multiple experimental groups with or without control group.
NS = Not significant.

Multicomponent programs address aspects of social learning theory (Bandura, 1971), including identification of cues to smoke, modification of one's environment, altering thought processes about smoking and withdrawal, relapse prevention techniques, and developing a reward system for nonsmoking behavior. Much of the attention focuses on an individualized plan to become a nonsmoker. Multicomponent treatment was used in almost half of the studies (Anthonisen et al., 1994; Burling et al., 1991; DeBusk et al., 1994; Hall et al., 1983; Hurt et al., 1994; Ockene et al., 1992; Pederson et al., 1991; Rigotti et al., 1994; Sawicki et al., 1993; Story & Stark, 1991; Taylor et al., 1990). Treatment ranged from a minimum of three face-to-face sessions to a maximum of 12 90-minute sessions delivered by nurses, health educators, lay counselors, or physicians.

Printed self-help material was frequently used to reinforce advice or multicomponent interventions (Ockene et al., 1992; Pederson et al., 1983; Pederson et al., 1991; Prue et al., 1983; Stevens et al., 1993), or it comprised the primary form of treatment (Rimer et al., 1994). Focus groups and survey data were used to develop *Clear Horizons,* a magazine-format intervention tailored to elderly smokers (Rimer et al., 1994). Another example was six bimonthly newsletters that supplemented smoking cessation begun with inpatients (Stevens et al., 1993).

Seven investigations incorporated telephone counseling as follow-up initiated by the researcher or as a hotline for persons to call for support (Anthonisen et al., 1994; DeBusk et al., 1994; Ockene et al., 1992; Prue et al., 1983; Rigotti et al., 1994; Rimer et al., 1994; Taylor et al., 1990). For example, Taylor et al. (1990) called persons weekly two or three times and then monthly four times; the Rimer and associates national study (1994) provided a hotline to an experimental group (n = 616).

Some treatments were used in only one or two studies. A videotape specific to inpatients was developed by Stevens and colleagues (1993); however, only 32% of those eligible actually viewed it. Two investigations included progressive muscle relaxation audiotapes (DeBusk et al., 1994; Taylor et al., 1990). Exercise and counseling were combined in two studies in which patients were in cardiac rehabilitation (Sivarajan et al., 1983; Taylor et al., 1988).

No studies of transdermal nicotine replacement met inclusion criteria for this review, however, nicotine gum was included in four studies (British Thoracic Society, 1983; Campbell et al., 1991; Anthonisen et al., 1994; Tønnesen et al., 1988). Significant treatment effect was reported in two investigations, although it is not possible to ascertain the effect of gum alone in these designs (Anthonisen et al., 1994; Tønnesen et al., 1988). Tønnesen and colleagues (1988) provided 2 mg and 4 mg of gum to individuals who received six 2-hour multicomponent sessions, compared to a control group of advice only and no nicotine replacement. Anthonisen et al. (1994) provided 2 mg of gum to nearly 4,000 participants, along with 12 intensive multicomponent sessions and an extensive maintenance period that included five meetings per year, quarterly newsletters, and regular telephone contact up to 5 years post-cessation. Nonsignificant treatment effect occurred in two studies (British Thoracic Society, 1983; Campbell et al., 1991). Experimental and control groups both received advice and 6-month follow-up support; 2 mg of gum and placebo were the distinguishing variables in the groups (Campbell et al., 1991). The British Thoracic Society (1983) study included four groups: (a) advice, (b) advice plus printed material, (c) same as (b) with placebo gum, (d) same as (b) with 2 mg of gum; they reported similar modest quit rates across the groups.

Severity of Comorbid Condition. Patients' perceptions about the severity of their comorbidity may have an impact on smoking cessation success. In persons with peripheral vascular disease, those with an aortic aneurysm diagnosis had a higher quit rate than individuals with intermittent claudication (50% vs. 25%, respectively). Ockene and associates (1992) found that smokers with: (a) documented acute myocardial infarction, (b) an arteriography after hospitalization, and (c) increased number of vessels involved had better cessation rates. However, Rigotti et al. (1994) reported no relationship between quit rate and severity of illness among patients following coronary artery bypass graft surgery. In one study (Sivarajan et al., 1983), 78% of those who quit cited acute myocardial infarction as the reason. In contradiction, a lower success rate was reported in those with self-reported chronic bronchitis, compared to their healthy counterparts (Tønnesen et al., 1988).

Smoking cessation interventions were applied less frequently in certain groups. A common misconception of lay persons and professionals is that it is "too late" for older smokers to quit, and thus fewer interventions are focused on the elderly (Rimer et al., 1994). A similar concern was expressed regarding individuals in substance abuse treatment, in that the stress of quitting smoking could jeopardize the abuser's recovery from substance abuse (Burling et al., 1991). However, there are no data to support this opinion, and in contrast, a smoking cessation program did not negatively affect the course of substance abuse therapy (Burling et al., 1991, Hurt et al., 1994).

Timing of the Intervention. Smokers hospitalized in a smoke-free environment present health professionals a window of opportunity for cessation instruction. Hospitalized patients who smoke are more likely to comply with cessation advice at the time of an acute illness (Schwartz, 1987). However, inpatients may receive limited smoking cessation information: 50% to 71% of smokers reported no advice to quit smoking during their hospital stays (Emmons & Goldstein, 1992; Goldstein, Westbrook, Howell, & Fischer, 1992). Interestingly, physicians and nurses on general medicine units intervened less frequently in this regard than did staff on a cardiovascular unit (Emmons & Goldstein, 1992). Several studies conducted with smokers who were diagnosed with cardiovascular disease (Campbell et al., 1991, DeBusk et al., 1994; Ockene et al., 1992; Rigotti et al., 1994; Taylor et al., 1990), pulmonary disease (Pederson et al., 1983; Pederson et al., 1991), head and neck cancer (Gritz et al., 1993), general medicine problems (Campbell et al., 1991; Stevens et al., 1993), substance abuse conditions (Burling et al., 1991), and alcohol abuse (Hurt et al., 1994) were initiated in an inpatient setting. Four of these studies reported significant improvement in quit rates at 6 or 12 months postintervention. The investigators have suggested that delivering the intervention while the smoker is hospitalized, in a smoke-free environment and often for a smoking-related disorder, improves receptivity to the cessation advice and counseling. Interestingly, for cardiovascular patients, interventions that were initiated during hospitalization were associated with higher success rates (DeBusk et al., 1994; Taylor et al., 1990), compared to those introduced only after discharge (Sivarajan et al., 1983; Taylor et al., 1988). With the exception of the nicotine replacement intervention studies among pulmonary patients (Anthonisen et al., 1994; Tønnesen et al., 1988), most outpatient studies have reported moderate success rates, ranging from 0% to 28% (Power et al., 1992; Prue et al., 1983; Sawicki et al., 1993; Story & Stark, 1991; Vetter & Ford, 1990).

Predictors of Cessation.   With regard to sociodemographic and smoking history variables, two studies (Campbell et al., 1991; Pederson et al., 1991) reported that older smokers are more apt to succeed; however, an earlier study by the same authors contradicted this finding (Pederson et al., 1983). Two studies have described male gender as a predictor of cessation (Ockene et al., 1992; Rimer et al., 1994), and one investigation reported no relationship between gender and quitting (Pederson et al., 1983). Rimer and others (1994) reported that more frequent serious attempts to quit, especially during the past year, improved cessation (odds ratio = 1.7). On the other hand, Rigotti et al. (1994) indicated that fewer than three previous attempts to quit was a significant predictor of abstinence (odds ratio = 7.4). Campbell et al. (1991) established that those who smoked between 16 and 25 cigarettes per day were more likely to succeed in quitting, compared to those who smoked more or fewer cigarettes each day. Pederson and others (1983) found no relationship between amount smoked and cessation. As expected, Ockene et al. (1992) and Gritz and associates (1993) both reported that participants in the action stage of smoking cessation were more likely to succeed in quitting.

Individuals' confidence in their ability to succeed at smoking cessation, or self-efficacy, would be related to successful quitting in a social learning theory framework (Bandura, 1971). Indeed, self-efficacy predicted or was related to success at 12 months in two investigations (Ockene et al., 1992;

Taylor et al., 1990). However, two-thirds of participants in the British Thoracic Society (1983) study stated that they were confident that they could quit smoking for at least 1 year, and quit rates at 6 months ranged from 9% to 11%. The effect of providers was evident when 76% of head and neck cancer participants recalled that their providers had expressed confidence in their ability to quit smoking (Gritz et al., 1993). Quit rates in intervention and control groups were 71% and 74% at 6 months, respectively, in the Gritz and associates study (1993).

Although not directly tested, an inpatient setting may facilitate cessation. Three studies have implied that longer, enforced hospital stays are associated with cessation (Campbell et al., 1991; Gritz et al., 1993; Stevens et al., 1993). As described above, this effect may also be related to timing of the intervention.

Several studies have reported equivocal results with regard to predictors of cessation. Although Rimer et al. (1994) reported that a desire to quit improved success rates, Pederson et al. (1991) was unable to establish a relationship between these variables. Likewise, two studies indicated that increased latency, or time to smoking the first cigarette of the day (a behavioral measure of dependence), was positively related to success (Gritz et al., 1993; Rimer et al., 1994); however, two studies found no relationship between time to first cigarette and successful cessation (Campbell et al., 1991; Tønnesen et al., 1988).

Other predictor variables reported to be associated with success in single studies included increased invasiveness of medical/surgical treatment (e.g., laryngectomy) (Gritz et al., 1993), advice by physician to stop smoking (Rimer et al., 1994), less reported dysphoria after cessation (Hall et al., 1983), use of multiple cessation strategies (Rimer et al., 1994), nonsmoking status at 3 weeks postintervention Taylor et al., 1990), and cessation 1 week prior to open heart surgery and no reported difficulty abstaining during the course of hospitalization (Rigotti et al., 1994).

DISCUSSION OF FINDINGS

As can be seen in Table 4.1, 7 of 23 studies reported a significant effect of treatment on smoking cessation (6 at 12 months and 1 at 6 months), and one study (Anthonisen et al., 1994) described a 25% improvement in quit rates with nicotine replacement but did not report the statistical analyses. As shown in Table 4.1, several studies reported significant but modest increases in the percentage of those who successfully quit smoking. These moderate rates are impressive if extrapolated to the adult smokers with comorbid conditions currently residing in the United States (Pierce et al., 1989).

Sample sizes in the studies with significant findings ranged from 101 to 5,887; seven of the eight studies included biochemical validation of smoking status by ECO_a or cotinine (Anthonisen et al., 1994; DeBusk et al., 1994; Hurt et al., 1994; Stevens et al., 1993; Taylor et al., 1990; Tønnesen et al., 1988; Vetter & Ford, 1990). Rimer et al. (1994) justified self-report as a measure of abstinence because of low-demand characteristics of the design with a national sample. Sample size was a factor in significance, as none of the 10 studies with fewer than 100 subjects was able to show a significant treatment effect.

These findings are promising and suggest that a variety of smoking cessation treatments are effective and can be used with groups of smokers with chronic illness. Individualized nurse-managed counseling interventions initiated during hospitalization, with extended outpatient follow-up, proved to be a highly effective form of treatment (DeBusk et al., 1994; Taylor et al., 1990; Vetter & Ford, 1990). Although the majority of nurses believe it is their responsibility to instruct patients about smoking cessation, the percentage who personally claim to counsel patients remains low (Faulkner, 1983; Sanders, 1986; Spencer, 1984). However, on the basis of the evidence, nurses represent competent smoking cessation interventionists.

Nicotine replacement therapy was associated with improved abstinence among those smokers diagnosed with pulmonary problems (Anthonisen et al., 1994; Tønnesen et al., 1988). Only one study examined nicotine replacement among smokers with cardiac diagnoses (Campbell et al., 1991), which may partially reflect cardiovascular patients' reluctance to use replacement therapy (Emmons & Goldstein, 1992).

Lack of distinct treatment differences across groups may have led to nonsignificant findings in several investigations with large sample sizes (British Thoracic Society, 1983; Campbell et al., 1991; Gritz et al., 1993; Sivarajan et al., 1983; Taylor et al., 1988). Although designs were experimental in nature, several investigators delivered minimal treatment, such as advice or printed pamphlets, to control groups. These low-intensity treatment methods may have been sufficient to prompt cessation, especially in selected groups (e.g., head and neck cancer).

DIRECTIONS FOR FUTURE RESEARCH

Although cessation interventions are being implemented with comorbid populations of smokers, the majority have been delivered to those with cardiovascular or pulmonary conditions. Little attention has been directed toward smokers diagnosed with cancer, diabetes, peripheral vascular diseases, substance abuse disorders, or toward elderly smokers. More research must be conducted to examine the effectiveness of cessation approaches among these groups. Similarly, most studies have involved well-educated male Caucasian smokers. Evaluation of treatment effects among diverse groups of smokers is indicated, especially in light of the projections for the year 2000, which forecast that a larger proportion of women (23%) than men (20%) will smoke, and more Blacks (25%) than Whites (21%) will engage in the behavior (Pierce et al., 1989). In addition, those who smoke will also represent the less educated.

Other important variables that deserve attention include (a) the stage of smoking cessation at initiation of treatment; (b) the influence of other dependent behaviors, such as alcohol, on successful abstinence; and (c) the contribution of significant others' smoking behavior to success in the presence of comorbidity. Also, information about the predictors of successful cessation is minimal and conflicting and requires further clarification. In addition, process evaluation during implementation would provide information regarding the actual effect of treatment, depending on the subjects' level of participation in assigned treatment.

Finally, the cost-effectiveness of cessation efforts has yet to be systematically addressed among comorbid populations. Only two studies (DeBusk et al., 1994; Tønnesen et al., 1988) directly discussed the cost of successful intervention. It has been reported that outpatient counseling against smoking is more cost-effective than other preventive health practices, such as treatment of mild to moderate hypertension or hypercholesterolemia (Cummings, Rubin, & Oster, 1989). As such, future investigators must delineate the cost-effectiveness of smoking cessation treatment in the presence of chronic illness.

REFERENCES

Achkar, E. (1985). Peptic ulcer disease: Current management in the elderly. *Geriatrics, 40*, 77–79.

Anthonisen, N. R., Connett, J. E., Kiley, J. P., Altose, M. D., Bailey, W. C., Buist, A. S., Conway, W. A., Enright, P. L., Kanner, R. E., O'Hara, P., Owens, G. P., Scanlon, P. D., Tashkin, D. P., Wise, R. A., for the Long Health Study Research Group. (1994). Effects of smoking intervention and the use of an inhaled anticholinergic bronchodilator on the rate of decline of FEV1. *Journal of the American Medical Association, 272*, 1497–1505.

Bandura, A. (1971). *Social learning theory*. Morristown, NJ: General Learning Press.

Benowitz, N. L. (1983). The use of biological fluid samples in assessing tobacco smoke consumption. In J. Grawbowski, & C. S. Bell (Eds.), *Measurement in the analysis and treatment of smoking behavior* (National Institute of Drug Abuse Research Monograph No. 48). Rockville, MD: National Institute of Drug Abuse.

Benowitz, N. L., Kuyt, F., Jacob, P., III, Jones, R. T., & Osman, A. L. (1983). Cotinine disposition and effects. *Clinical Pharmacology and Therapeutics, 34*, 604–611.

Bloom, R. J., Stevick, C. A., & Lemmon, S. (1990). Patient perspectives on smoking a peripheral vascular disease: A veteran survey population. *American Surgeon, 56*, 535–539.

British Thoracic Society. (1983). Comparison of four methods of smoking withdrawal in patients with smoking related diseases. *British Medical Journal, 286*, 595–597.

Burling, T. A., Marshall, G. D., & Seidner, A. L. (1991). Smoking cessation for substance abuse inpatients. *Journal of Substance Abuse, 3*, 269–276.

Campbell, I. A., Prescott, R. J., & Tjeder-Burton, S. M. (1991). Smoking cessation in hospital patients given repeated advice plus nicotine or placebo chewing gum. *Respiratory Medicine, 85*, 155–157.

Centers for Disease Control. (1991). Cigarette smoking among adults—United States. *Morbidity and Mortality Weekly Review, 42*, 230–233.

Cummings, S. R., Rubin, S. M., & Oster, G. (1989). The cost-effectiveness of counseling smokers to quit. *Journal of the American Medical Association, 261*, 75–79.

DeBusk, R. F., Miller, N. H., Superko, H. R., Dennis, C. A., Thomas, R. J., Lew, H. T., Berger, W. E., Heller, R. S, Rompf, J., & Gee, D. (1994). A case-management system for coronary risk factor modification after acute myocardial infarction. *Annals of Internal Medicine, 120*, 721–729.

DeSoto, C. B., O'Donnell, W. E., & DeSoto, J. L. (1989). Long-term recovery in alcoholics. *Alcoholism: Clinical and Experimental Research, 13*, 693–697.

Emmons, K. M., & Goldstein, M. G. (1992). Smokers who are hospitalized: A window of opportunity for cessation interventions. *Preventive Medicine, 21*, 262–269.

Fisher, E. B., Haire-Joshu, D., Morgan, G. D., Rehberg, H., & Rost, K. (1990). Smoking and smoking cessation. *American Review of Respiratory Disease, 142*, 702–720.

Faulkner, A. (1983). Nurses as health educators in relation to smoking. *Nursing Times, 79*, 47–48.

Goldstein, A. O., Westbrook, W. R., Howell, R. E., & Fischer, P. M. (1992). Hospital efforts in smoking control: Remaining barriers and challenges. *Journal of Family Practice, 34*, 729–734.

Gritz, E. R., Carr, C. R., Rapkin, D., Abemayor, E., Chang, L J., Wong, W. K., Beumer, J., & Ward, P. H. (1993). Predictors of long-term smoking cessation in head and neck cancer patients. *Cancer Epidemiology Biomarkers and Prevention, 2*, 261–270.

Hall, S. M., Bachman, J., Henderson, J. B., Barstow, R., & Jones, R. T. (1983). Smoking cessation in patients with cardiopulmonary disease: An initial study. *Addictive Behaviors, 8*, 33–42.

Hurt, R. D., Eberman, K. M., Croghan, I. T., Offord, K. P., Davis, L. J., Morse, R. M., Palmer, M. A., & Bruce, K. A. (1994). Nicotine dependence treatment during inpatient treatment for other addictions: A prospective intervention trial. *Alcoholism, Clinical and Experimental Research, 18*, 867–872.

Jarvis, M. J., Tunstall-Pedoe, H., Feyerabend, C., Vesey, C., & Saloojee, Y. (1984). Biochemical markers of smoke absorption and self-reported exposure to passive smoking. *Journal of Epidemiology and Community Health, 38*, 335–339.

McIntyre-Kingsolver, K. O., Lichtenstein, E., & Mermelstein, R. J. (1983). Spouse training in a multicomponent smoking-cessation program. *Journal of Consulting and Clinical Psychology, 51*, 632–633.

Mellstrom, D., Rundgren, A., Jagenburg, R., Steen, B., & Svanborg, A. (1982). Tobacco smoking, aging and health among the elderly: A longitudinal study of 70 year old men and an age cohort comparison. *Age and Aging, 11*, 45–48.

Mulhauser, I., Sawicki, P., & Berger, M. (1986). Cigarette-smoking as a risk factor for macroproteinuria and proliferative retinopathy in type 1 (insulin-dependent) diabetes. *Diabetologia, 29*, 500–502.

Ockene, J. K., Benfari, R. C., Nuttall, R. L., Hurwitz, I., & Ockene I. S. (1982). Relationship of psychosocial factors to smoking behavior change in an intervention program. *Preventive Medicine, 11*, 13–28.

Ockene, J. K., Kristeller, J. L., Goldberg, R., Ockene, I., Merriam, P., Barrett, S., Pekow, P., Hosmer, D., & Gianelly, R. (1992). Smoking cessation and severity of disease: The Coronary Artery Intervention Study. *Health Psychology, 11*, 119–126.

Pederson, L. L., Lefcoe, N. M., & Wood, T. (1983). Use of a self-help smoking cessation manual as an adjunct to advice from a respiratory specialist. *International Journal of the Addictions, 18*, 777–782.

Pederson, L. L., Wanklin, J. M., & Lefcoe, N. M. (1991). The effects of counseling on smoking cessation among patients hospitalized with chronic obstructive pulmonary disease. *International Journal of the Addictions, 26*, 107–119.

Pierce, J. P., Fiore, M. C., Novotny, T. E., Hatziandreu, E. J., & Davis, R. M. (1989). Trends in cigarette smoking in the United States projections to the year 2000. *Journal of the American Medical Association, 261*, 61–65.

Power, L., Brown, N. S., & Makin, G. S. (1992). Unsuccessful outpatient counselling to help patients with peripheral vascular disease to stop smoking. *Annals of the Royal College of Surgeons of England, 74*, 31–34.

Prochaska, J., & DiClemente, C. (1983). Stages and processes of self-change of smoking: Toward an integrative model of change. *Journal of Consulting and Clinical Psychology, 51*, 390–395.

Prochaska, J. (1992). A transtheoretical model of behavior change: Learning from mistakes with majority populations. In D. M. Becker, D. R. Hill, J. S. Jackson, D. M. Levine, F. Stillman, & S. M. Weiss (Eds.), *Health behavior research in minority populations: Access, design and implementation.* (DDHS Publication No. 92-2965). Washington, DC: U.S. Government Printing Office.

Prue, D. M., Davis, C. J., Martin, J. E., & Moss, R. A. (1983). An investigation of a minimal contact brand fading program for smoking treatment. *Addictive Behaviors, 8*, 307–310.

Richardson, G. E., Tucker, M. A., Venson, D. J., Linnoila, R. I., Phelps, R., Phares, J. C., Edison, M., Inde, D. C., & Johnson, B. E. (1993). Smoking cessation after successful treatment of small-cell lung cancer is associated with fewer smoking-related second primary cancers. *Annals of Internal Medicine, 119*, 383–390.

Rigotti, N. A., McKool, K. M., & Shiffman, S. (1994). Predictors of smoking cessation after coronary artery bypass graft surgery: Results of a randomized trial with 5-year follow-up. *Annals of Internal Medicine, 120*, 287–293.

Rimer, B. K., Orleans, C. T., Fleisher, L., Cristinzio, S., Resch, N., Telepchak, J., & Keintz, M. K. (1994). Does tailoring matter? The impact of a tailored guide on ratings and short-term smoking-related outcomes for older smokers. *Health Education Research, 9*, 69–84.

Sanders, D. (1986). Practice nurses and antismoking education. *British Medical Journals, 292*, 381–384.

Sawicki, P. T., Didjurgeit, U., Muhlhauser, I., & Berger, M. (1993). Behaviour therapy versus doctor's anti-smoking advice in diabetic patients. *Journal of Internal Medicine, 234*, 407–409.

Schwartz, J. S. (1987). *Review and evaluation of smoking cessation methods: The United States and Canada, 1978-1985* (NIH Publication 87-2940). Washington, DC: U.S. Government Printing Office.

Shiffman, S. (1979). The tobacco withdrawal syndrome (National Institute of Drug Abuse Research Monograph No. 23: 158-184). Rockville, MD: National Institute of Drug Abuse.

Sivarajan, E. S., Newton, K. M., Almes, M. J., Kempf, T. M., & Bruce, R. A. (1983). The patient after myocardial infarction: Limited effects of outpatient teaching and counseling after myocardial infarction: A controlled study. *Heart and Lung, 12*, 65–73.

Somerville, K., Faulkner, G., & Langman, M. (1986). Non-steroidal anti-inflammatory drugs and bleeding peptic ulcer. *Lancet, 1*, 462–464.

Spencer, J. (1984). Nurses' cigarette smoking in England and Wales. *International Journal of Nursing Studies, 21*, 69–79.

Stevens, V. J., Glasgow, R. E., Hollis, J. F., Lichtenstein, E., & Vogt, T. M. (1993). A smoking-cessation intervention for hospital patients. *Medical Care, 31*, 65–72.

Story, J., & Stark, M. J. (1991). Treating cigarette smoking in methadone maintenance clients. *Journal of Psychoactive Drugs, 23*, 203–215.

Taylor, C. B., Houston-Miller, N., Haskell, W. L., & DeBusk, R. F. (1988). Smoking cessation after acute myocardial infarction: The effects of exercise training. *Addictive Behaviors, 13*, 331–335.

Taylor, C. B., Houston-Miller, N., Killen, J. D., & DeBusk, R. F. (1990). Smoking cessation after acute myocardial infarction: Effects of a nurse-managed intervention. *Annals of Internal Medicine, 113*, 118–123.

Tønnesen, P., Fryd, V., Hansen, M., Helsted, J., Gunnerson, A. B., Forchammer, H., & Stockner, M. (1988). Two and four mg nicotine chewing gum and group counselling in smoking cessation: An open, randomized, controlled trial with a 22 month follow-up. *Addictive Behaviors, 13*, 17–27.

U.S. Department of Health and Human Services. (1988). *The health consequences of smoking: Nicotine addiction. A report of the surgeon general* (DHHS Publication No. CDC 88-8406). Washington, DC: U.S. Government Printing Office.

U.S. Department of Health and Human Services. (1989). *Reducing the health consequences of smoking: 25 years of progress: A report of the Surgeon General* (DHHS Publication No. CDC 89-8411). Washington, DC: U.S. Government Printing Office.

U.S. Department of Health and Human Services. (1990a). *The health benefits of smoking cessation: A report of the surgeon general* (DHHS Publication No. CDC 90-8416). Washington, DC: U.S. Government Printing Office.

U.S. Department of Health and Human Services. (1990b). *Healthy people 2000: National health promotion and disease objectives* (DHHS Publication No. 91-50213). Washington, DC: U.S. Government Printing Office.

Velicer, W. F., Prochaska, J. O., Rossi, J. S., & Snow, M. G. (1992). Assessing outcome in smoking cessation studies. *Psychological Bulletin, 111*, 23–41.

Vetter, N. J., & Ford, D. (1990). Smoking prevention among people aged 60 and over: A randomized controlled trial. *Age and Aging, 19*, 164–168.

Chapter 5

Quality of Life and Caregiving in Technological Home Care

CAROL E. SMITH

SCHOOL OF NURSING

UNIVERSITY OF KANSAS

CONTENTS

Technological home care has been described as a system of health services delivered by families who manage the care at home of individuals dependent on technology for survival (Andre, 1986; Copeman & Weigel, 1987; Lange, 1986; C. E. Smith, 1995). This chapter followed "Technology and Home Care" of the *Annual Review of Nursing Research* (Vol. 13), which focused on the efficacy, cost-effectiveness, and delivery of home services of the six most commonly used technologies. This second chapter describes in detail the quality-

95

of-life responses to technological dependence and the challenges that families face in caregiving, becoming educated in technological care, and managing costs associated with technological home care.

Research cited herein was identified through computerized searches (MEDLINE, Psycholiterature [PsychLIT], Cumulative Index to Nursing and Allied Health Literature [CINAHL], using the terms quality of life, family caregivers, ethical issues, home care, and guidelines/standards of care. The names of the most common technologies used for long-term survival were also used in the search. Research from various disciplines from 1975 to 1994 was retrieved and included in the review if subjects in the study were patients, family members, or caregivers managing home technology care and if the study focused on issues related to quality of life. Historical endeavors that have influenced research in the area, such as congressional directives, consensus conferences, and international reports, are cited.

The federal Office of Technology Assessment (OTA) defines someone as technologically dependent when he or she needs a medical device to compensate for the loss of a vital body function and also requires ongoing nursing care from either a lay person or a professional to avert death or further disability (U.S. Congress, OTA, 1987a). Technologies meeting this definition include mechanical ventilation, parenteral nutrition, hemodialysis or peritoneal dialysis, infusion therapies, external cardioverter devices, and cardiac/respiratory electronic monitoring. Spouses, parents, or significant others are the main providers of home care; thus, it is essential to understand their needs and other family members' responses related to technological dependency.

HOME CARE TECHNOLOGIES

Efficacy and reliability of technology, availability of home care services, cost control measures, and growth in public or consumer demands for life-sustaining care have resulted in a growing population of technologically dependent adults and children at home (C. E. Smith, 1995). Although government documents warn that data on the numbers of technologically dependent individuals are difficult to ascertain, Medicare figures and home care industry reports have been used to extrapolate estimates. Annually, there are approximately 4,000 to 6,000 adults and 2,000 to 3,000 children at home requiring mechanical ventilation, 7,000 to 45,000 children and a greater number of adults requiring apnea monitoring and/or oxygen assist devices, 40,000 patients on parenteral and enteral nutrition, 3,000 on hemodialysis, and 4,000 (mostly children) on continuous ambulatory peritoneal dialysis (CAPD). There are also thousands estimated to require automatic external cardiac defibrillation for life-threatening cardiac arrhythmias. Millions of others need home intravenous infusions (for medications, immunoglobins, chemotherapy, or epidural analgesia) with potential for growth as the new Medicare regulations reimburse for home antibiotic therapy for elders. Each of these therapies has been found to be cost-effective and safe when undertaken in the home. But extensive use also has challenged families' quality of life and has raised other questions.

In 1984, congressional committees on aging instigated a national study of medical technologies that sustain life to answer "new questions about quality of life," roles of families, financial barriers, and ethical dilemmas concerning decisions made by technologically dependent patients, their families, and health care practitioners. In response to this request, the OTA awarded contracts for studying the efficacy of five technologies (mechanical ventilation, hemodialysis, parenteral and enteral nutritional support/hydration, life-sustaining antibiotic therapy, and cardiopulmonary resuscitation) and used advisory panels of experts and consumers to establish guidelines for technology use (U.S. Congress, OTA, 1987a, 1987b). In addition, background papers from six other countries were generated that described systems of care, including home management of technologically dependent persons. The OTA established groundwork for legislative policy. Consensus conferences on withholding and withdrawing mechanical ventilation were held, and guidelines were published in 1987. These guidelines have affected clinical practice and are now considered when long-term technological dependence is being considered. Specifically, the guidelines take into account the person's right to choose care, the severity of the illness, the family caregiver's ability to manage home care, and the potential for quality of life in the technologically dependent person and the family members.

QUALITY OF LIFE WITH HOME CARE TECHNOLOGY

Studies that were focused on quality of life across all technological areas historically relied on patient functional status, illness parameters, and longevity as indicators of quality. Recently, indicators have been expanded to include patient and family members' perceptions of well-being. The initial studies in which researchers used an economic theoretical perspective (entitled utility assessment) helped establish technology treatment efficacy. Utility assessment results in a Quality Adjusted Life Years rating score of the patient's health state, calculated as the number of years of additional survival (Torrance, 1987; Torrance, Boyle, & Horwood, 1982; Weinstein, 1983).

Nutrition Support and Quality of Life

One quality of life study using utility assessment of 73 patients receiving home-infused total parenteral nutrition (TPN) in Toronto, Canada, indicated an average 3.3 years of additional survival, improved health, and cost savings of

$19,232 per patient (Detsky et al., 1986). In spite of stabilization of patients' nutrition status by TPN and reported returns to normal lifestyles, they indicated that social restrictions (Ladefoged, 1980), not having portable infusion pumps (Boutin & Hagan, 1992), fatigue, and worry over finances decreased life satisfaction (Smith, 1993). Researchers using standardized measures have consistently pointed out that long-term TPN patients report lower quality of life, compared to healthy populations (Herfindal, Bernstein, Kudzia, & Wong, 1989; C. E. Smith, 1993). Controversy over the use of TPN in clinical populations where quality of life and survival are doubtful (e.g., chemotherapy, terminal cancer, or AIDS) is based on conflicting research findings on the efficacy of nutrition support (American College of Physicians, 1989; Howard, 1992; Klein, Simes, & Blackburn, 1986; Mattox, 1993; Singer et al., 1991). Ethical issues related to withdrawal of food and, particularly, hydration have been discussed extensively but not necessarily in relation to home care technology (Knox, 1989). In the TPN studies, although different measurement instruments have been used, the research focus on quality of life has expanded beyond survival data to include patient and family perceptions. Conceptual dimensions and measures of life quality have been broadened and aligned with classic research in the field of quality of life.

Ventilation and Quality of Life

Splaingard, Frates, Harrison, Carter, and Jefferson (1983) used a life-table analysis that indicates a 3-year increased survival of the majority of 26 adults and 21 children using positive-pressure ventilation at home. In another study of life-table analysis of 54 children requiring home ventilation, researchers followed families longitudinally. They found that there were no significant differences between number of deaths in patients using nurses 24 hours per day in the home and those with family care alone (Frates, Splaingard, Smith, & Harrison, 1985). In this study, 2 of 54 children were eventually transferred to nursing home care, at 3 and 14 years, respectively, because parents could no longer manage home care.

Currently, ventilator-dependent patients live well beyond the survival rates in the early 1980 studies, although technical side effects create psychological distress (C. E. Smith, Faust-Wilson, Lohr, Kallenberger, & Marien, 1992). Families report some quality in their lives, but they say it is affected by the limitations technology brings to the child's growth and development. Specifically, lowered self-esteem and anxiety associated with self-rejection and depression have been reported in technologically dependent children due to overprotection by parents. Factors associated with the child's autonomy included family and peer support, involvement with household duties, and having friends with and without disabilities.

The economic strain on the household also decreases quality of life. Studies of ventilator-dependent children in numerous states have verified that finances and out-of-pocket expenses are major factors that increase strain on families (Millner, 1991; Motwani & Herring, 1988; Wegener & Aday, 1989). Prior to a 1984 waiver, Medicaid did not allow payment for children on technological home care. Funding allowing such home care for children required substantial copayments that would have reduced most families to the poverty level (Foundation for Hospice and Homecare, 1987; U.S. Congress, OTA, 1987b). Logically, conceptualizations of quality of life must be expanded to encompass these important issues.

Dialysis and Quality of Life

In a large multisite hemodialysis center comparison using national probability sampling ($N = 859$), R. W. Evans and colleagues (1985) found home hemodialysis patients had higher quality-of-life scores than did CAPD patients. This study moved beyond survival as a measure of quality of life by using objective measures of employment and functional capacity as well as three subjective measures (life satisfaction, well-being, and psychological effect). These measures had been found valid and reliable in other studies of technologically dependent and chronically ill adults. As other researchers indicated, scores from Evans's dialysis patients were lower than those of healthy adults (Eschbach, Egrie, Downing, Browne, & Adamson, 1987; E. Fox et al., 1991; Simmons & Abress, 1990; Simmons, Anderson, & Kamstra, 1984; Winearls et al., 1986).

In a matched convenience sample, both CAPD and hemodialysis patients reported that perceived health was related to quality of life (Bihl, Ferrans, & Powers, 1988). DeKeyser (1990) identified a weak relationship between peritoneal immune function and psychosocial measures of stress, anxiety, and depression in 32 CAPD patients. A significant inverse correlation existed between the number of children treated at a specialized CAPD center and peritonitis risk, indicating a possible relationship between the type of treatment experienced and reduced patient side effects, including greatly enhanced quality of life (Alexander, Lindbad, Nolph, & Novach, 1990). Accusations of bias based on race or socioeconomic level in determining dialysis treatment (center or home dialysis) and renal transplant recipients have been made, but they have not been verified by large-scale studies (M. Smith, Hang, Michelman, & Robson, 1983). Hart and Evans (1987) argued that differences in medical management, treatment modalities, and quality-of-life outcomes, such as sleep, rest, work, and recreation, are not associated with home care but result from patient age and comorbidity variations.

Molzahn (1991) conducted a qualitative study on quality of life based on the Aristotelian-Thomistic philosophical theory in 10 home hemodialysis patients. All patients were rated as having the means and possessions for good lives, although political liberty, defined as equal opportunity for employment, was compromised. According to the Aristotelian-Thomistic theory, these patients had compromised quality of life, whereas atheoretical research could have overlooked the employment dimension of life quality. This study, although using a theory typically applied at the group or community level, provided insights into families' concern over employment hindrances.

Infusion and Quality of Life

In areas of infusion technology that facilitate long-term treatments at home that are needed for survival, few studies of quality of life have been conducted. A series of studies on intravenous immunoglobulin given by family caregivers has verified the difficulties of but also the preference for this home therapy. The measure of quality of life correlated positively with the psychological benefits of home-based intravenous immunoglobulin infusion therapy (J. H. Evans, Daly, Kobayashi, & Kobayashi, 1988). Payne (1992) reported that the quality of life of 53 patients with advanced breast or ovarian cancer, who were on home chemotherapy, was higher than for patients receiving hospital-administered therapy.

Suicide by withdrawal of technology has been reported (Roberts & Kjellstrand, 1988), and this issue was discussed in an Institute of Medicine report (Rettig & Levinsky, 1991). Withdrawal of technology or technological failure and the associated human factors and deaths are under study by the Committee on Human Factors, National Research Council, and the National Academy of Science (1995).

The overall knowledge gained from studies of the technology-dependent individual was that the quality of life was acceptable to the vast majority of patients studied. However, much of the research was conducted without a theoretical or conceptual basis related to quality of life and was measured by a variety of techniques and instruments that limited comparisons. Contrasts from studies of children and adults highlight the need to consider the patients' developmental levels and the impact of the technological dependence on life tasks and goals.

Quality-of-life definitions should be more broadly defined to include the patient and family measures of productive social life (Benner, 1985). In 1989 the Institute of Medicine published a monograph titled *Quality of Life and Technology Assessment.* Various instruments that focused on physical, psychological, family, and social-economic aspects of quality-of-life measurement were identified. The use of theory-based psychometrically sound instruments will more accurately convey the experiences of technologically dependent patients and their family caregivers.

FAMILY CAREGIVING WITH HOME CARE TECHNOLOGIES

The problems disrupting quality of life that are commonly reported by care-givers who provide technological care include burdens of physical care, financial strain, and difficulty in coping with individual role and schedule disruption (Bergstrom, 1986; Kuhn,1980; Lindgren, 1987; C. E. Smith, Fernengel, Werkowitz, & Holcroft, 1992). Also identified as problems are the stress of learning to manage the technology, the unavailability of community medical care resources, accepting help from others, and observing negative changes in the patient (Corby, Schad, & Fudge, 1986; Davis, 1980; Miller, 1985). Other problems noted include depression, social isolation, anxiety, and the need for home remodeling (C. E. Smith, Mayer, Parkhurst, Perkins, & Pingleton, 1991; C. E. Smith, Moushey, Ross, & Geifer, 1993).

Problems of families managing technologically dependent children at home have been studied in several states. Focus group interviews were used to collect data from 80 parents of technologically dependent children across the state of Florida. Recurrent themes from these interviews were the need for organization of services for access and coordination of assistance. Lack of services, training, information, equipment, financial assistance, and ability to plan for the future (whether for the child's education or death) were discussed (Diehl, Moffitt, & Wade, 1991).

Families surveyed across the state of New York expressed difficulties with cash flow and deciphering home care service charges and relationships between multiple payor sources (Motwani & Herring, 1988). Local primary care physicians and community resources such as emergency services and adaptable school systems were often lacking. Continuity of care was monitored after discharge but not formally by a multidisciplinary team (Goldberg, et al., 1987; Plummer, O'Donohue, & Petty, 1989). Other issues raised in consensus groups and in research findings were the difficulties in starting withdrawal from the technology when the patient's quality of life deteriorated and nurses' ambivalence about this withdrawal process (Bayer, 1987; Daly, Newlon, Montenegro, & Langdon, 1993; Fry, 1990).

Only one early study was oriented toward describing factors that contributed to successful caregiving in home technology care. Stiller (1988) conducted a retrospective chart review by using nurses' ratings. Two groups of families emerged from the nurses' ratings of family coping. The "unsuccessful" group of seven families had low family coping scores and more frequent problems, such as lack of compliance, fatigue of caregivers, and mental or emotional problems of either patient or caregiver. The "successful" group (12 families) had high family coping index scores and infrequent problems. The two groups were similar on medical prognosis of the patient, insurance coverage, types of technology used, and the mean number (4) of nursing visits required for families

to learn the procedures of home care. Stiller concluded that when the wife/ mother was the patient and a male caregiver assumed new responsibilities, there was less family coping than when the caregiver was female. Stiller emphasized that family coping ability, not the demands of high-technology care, accounted for caregiver success in managing home care. In descriptive studies of patients on home technology, researchers frequently have made inferences about the importance of the family caregivers. However, few studies have been focused specifically on caregivers.

Caregiving for Oxygen-Dependent Patients

In an attempt to identify caregivers at risk of experiencing stress from home care, a cross-sectional prospective study was conducted with 121 parents of ventilator-dependent children (Wegener & Aday, 1989). Two standardized Likert-type instruments were used, the Family Impact Scale to measure stress of living with a chronically ill child and the Caregiver Well-Being Scale to measure frequency of stress symptoms. None of the child's characteristics (prognosis, number of other illnesses, hours on ventilator per day) was a significant predictor. This was interpreted by researchers as indicating that even the most severely ill child with the greatest dependence on ventilation per day can be managed at home. The variables that did contribute to family and caregiver stress, however, were finances (viewed as serious monetary problems, increased out-of-pocket expenses), a single-parent household, lack of extended family to aid the caregiver, lack of continuity of care (patients required to see multiple physicians and no nurse case manager), and a noncomprehensive discharge plan. Home ventilation problems include increased long-term family stress and financial strain from costs not covered by third-party payors, such as the need to remodel homes to accommodate ventilation equipment, electrical bills, supplies, portable ventilators, and special transportation needs for the patient (Lobosco, Eron, Bobo, Kril, & Chalenick, 1991). These data were used to influence policy for long-term availability of case management nurses and to provide practice guidelines for financial assessment and comprehensive discharge planning.

Longitudinal studies of caregivers of adult ventilator patients indicated that as caregivers became more experienced, their needs changed from concerns about emergency care to wanting financial and respite care information (Thomas, Ellison, Howell, & Winters, 1992). Longitudinal prospective studies of differing caregiving situations in families with different developmental levels are needed (Gipson, Sivak, & Gulledge, 1987; C. E. Smith, Mayer, et al., 1991). Overall, these correlational descriptive studies of caregivers indicated that life improves when the patient comes home because of increased commu-

nication and family problem-solving, resumption of nearly normal everyday activities, and a sense of confidence from managing home care.

Geary (1989) identified 10 themes after interviewing 20 women who cared for full-term infants requiring oxygen and home apnea monitoring. Geary concluded that the intensity of the theme "managing the monitor" suggests mothers had little energy left for other activities. Sweeney (1988) found no mood disturbance differences between mothers of apnea-monitored and non-apnea-monitored infants at 3 months postdischarge. However, mood disturbance scores of men (other-parent caretakers) were lower than those of mothers in both groups. These studies had the advantage of being prospective and longitudinal, thus providing evidence of the ongoing and dynamic needs of caregiving over time.

Caregiving for Nutrition-Supported Patients

In 1990 the Department of Health and Human Services provided a contract for the Program on Technology and Health Care of the Georgetown University School of Medicine to convene a forum to establish guidelines for appropriate use of TPN, based on safety, effectiveness, and cost. The forum members assessed the state of knowledge regarding use of TPN in various clinical populations, enumerated the safety concerns, described economic analysis and cost-control strategies, discussed the legal/ethical issues, and developed practice guidelines for clinical decision making. The recommendations for practice guidelines, costs, safety, and ethical issues were based on a review of research in the area. However, forum members noted that no data from prospective randomized studies existed on home parenteral nutrition patients at that time. Quality of life was only anecdotally reported.

A model based on the Roy Adaptation framework guided two studies of family adaptation to a patient's technological dependency in the home (C. E. Smith, Giefer, & Bieker, 1991). The model, depicting self-care practices and adaptation to high-technology home care, was pilot-tested in a study of five rural families living 50 miles from durable-equipment companies that supply infusion material. In the first few months at home, caregivers reported anxiety about learning the technological care, lack of control related to machine dependency, and depression, even though the family members rated themselves as adapting well. In a study of an urban sample of TPN-dependent patients, caregivers' depression and anxiety were commonly identified as problems, although the family caregivers rated themselves as adapting well on a family adaptation instrument (C. E. Smith, Moushey, Ross, & Giefer, 1993). Difficulties with caregiving (daily schedule disruption, negative reactions, resentment, patient health deterioration) and anxiety were associated with depression but not with caregivers' physical health. Social stigma or isolation were problematic for many families, and financial strain was almost universal. A prospective national study, with 178 randomly selected pairs of caregivers and TPN-dependent patients was based on these reports (C. E. Smith, 1993). The study confirmed that caregivers' family coping, mutuality in the dyad relationship, and motivation for caregiving were positively associated with their quality of life. Depression, financial strain, and length of time of caregiving were negatively associated.

Spouses of 172 adults dependent on home TPN were surveyed by means of an 8-item ranking mailed questionnaire (Heaphy, 1988). Depression, control or independence issues, and relationship with spouse were ranked as the most significant problems by both patients and caregivers. Yet when asked to list and rank the most important resources of help with psychosocial problems, the spouse was rated as number 1. Caregivers indicated that body image distortion and sexual difficulties were resolved, whereas patients ranked these problems as significant. These findings highlighted the differences in the patients' and spouse/caregivers' reactions to home TPN. Preliminary studies, followed by larger samples with more comprehensive data on common and sensitive issues, provided a clear description of the impact of home care on the caregiver. However, little information on other family members has been reported.

Caregiving for Dialysis-Dependent Patients

In an early study of preparing families for home hemodialysis, Fishman and Schneider (1972) reported that patients and their caregivers' long-term emotional adjustments at 1 year were related to problem-solving ability. Bryan and Evans (1980), in a national survey of 1,198 home dialysis patients and their caregivers, found that 92% of caregivers knew they could make mistakes or experience machine problems, but these thoughts did not worry them. In addition, 80.8% of respondents stated they reduced outside activities to give care. In another study, distress scores of spouses of hospital versus home dialysis patients did not differ; however, home spouses reported fewer social problems (Soskolne & DeNour, 1987). In a prospective study of 32 patients on home dialysis and 29 spouses, depression, anxiety, and marital problems were encountered less frequently when spouses were trained as assistants rather than as sole providers of the treatment (Lowry & Atcherson, 1980), even though spouses report assisting each dialysis infusion (Rydholm & Pauling, 1991).

Investigators observing families indicated that home dialysis can lead to family unhappiness, deterioration in standard of living (Hatz & Powers, 1980), excessive marital closeness, submergence of caregiver needs, and control

exercised by the dialysis patient over family members (Palmer, Canzona, & Wai, 1982). Peterson (1985) studied the psychosocial adjustment of female family caregivers and concluded that family financial resources, patient physical and emotional status, and the caregiver's work history interact to impact the caregiver's adjustment. Because the sample size was small and the caregiver's adjustment was measured by a staff nurse's rating, Peterson's conclusions need to be interpreted cautiously. In contrast, Gurklis and Menke (1988) found situational factors such as age, severity of patient condition, suddenness of onset, and length of time of technological dependence were associated with coping mechanisms used by caregivers and patients (Gonsalves-Ebrahim, Sterin, Gulledge, Gipson, & Rodgers, 1987). Srivastava (1988) indicated that the coping strategies most often used with dialysis patients and caregivers may not be those that are most effective for adaptation. The home dialysis population is possibly the most extensively studied, yet generalizations of findings are not possible because the financial demands of expensive technology and out-of-pocket expenses are not present in this population with federally paid health care.

The emphasis of these descriptive caregiving studies has been on identifying the problems and difficulties experienced by family members of technologically dependent persons. However, caregiver and patient data and home care workers' observations suggested the overwhelming desire to keep the patient on technology and at home. Compared to hospital care, a greater sense of control and positive morale have been reported by both family members and patients on home technological care as a result of the resumption of more normal interactions and routines of daily living (Frace, 1986; Goldberg, 1983).

Few studies have been longitudinal or have been focused on transitions in caregiving, such as the effects of the caregiver's becoming ill, the patient's being rehospitalized, or the inability of extended family or friends to assist with home care. Also, comparisons have not been made between caregiving demands of differing home technologies.

Research on families managing technology in the home must turn to quality-of-life issues that are germane to the elderly and also to culturally diverse populations (King, Figge, & Jarman, 1986; Roy, Flynn, & Atcherson, 1980). Although ethnicity and gender were reported in many studies, only a few samples analyzed or discussed data relative to these perspectives or characteristics (Guilleminault, Quera-Salva, Partinen, & Jamieson, 1988).

Ethical issues of patient care, like being abandoned or abused by caregivers or caregiving obligations overriding caregivers' quality of life, were recently studied in a *Hastings Center Report* (Arras, 1994) titled "Technological Tether: When the Hospital Goes Home." Families need counseling and education in these areas.

PATIENT EDUCATION WITH HOME CARE TECHNOLOGIES

Research on patient education indicated that preparation for discharge can ease the transition from hospital to home. Pediatric discharge preparations for aiding transition to home technological care have been tested (Barnard et al., 1987; Kruger & Rawlins, 1984). Steele and Harrison (1986) tested a protocol whereby parents of ventilator-assisted children were trained for home care by providing 24-hour total care in hospital prior to discharge. The protocol included a signed contract between parents and a nurse case manager. All six families (including a single parent) were evaluated as successful. In this study success was defined as home care, with minimal intervention from professional staff, being implemented within 3 days to 2 weeks of the in-hospital trial. A byproduct of the signed contract was more effective collaboration between health care workers themselves.

Goldstein (1991) verified hypotheses that patients going home with right atrial infusion catheters, together with their family members, had greater learning outcomes (demonstration of skills and knowledge) and fewer rehospitalizations for catheter complications at 3 months when taught in a hospital learning center prior to discharge. The learning center was described as a laboratory where central venous access device simulators and mannequins were available, and practice/demonstrations were overseen by registered nurses. Home health nurses who rated families' postdischarge preparation indicated that, compared to routine hospital discharge, it took less time per visit and patients were less nervous when they had been taught in the center.

Thompson and Richmond (1990) ascertained that 13 home ventilator adult patients perceived that discharge planning should be offered in the hospital with family members present. C. E. Smith, Mayer, Perkins, Gerald, and Pingleton (1994) recommended a staged teaching program based on the results of a survey of learning needs from caregivers of home ventilator patients. Caregivers reported positive attitudes toward health care workers who had taught them home ventilator care, but they also indicated their desire to learn from other caregivers in similar circumstances.

National reports indicate that 2% of hospital readmissions are due to a need to reeducate caregivers and TPN-dependent patients [OLEY/A.S.P.E.N. Information System (OASIS 1987)]. Although no comparison group was used, children who had read an educational booklet about TPN were reported to have less anxiety (Laine et al., 1988). In a case study, Lansky, Doerr, and Ivey (1982) successfully taught TPN home management to an adult with limited mentation. Caregivers of TPN-dependent patients rated educational content about physical and technical care as satisfactorily taught but noted that information on social-emotional aspects of adjusting to home was not adequately provided (C. E. Smith, Moushey, Marien, & Weber, 1993).

Home training for hemodialysis and CAPD have been studied since inception (Atcherson & Lowry, 1981; Jeffrey, Heidenheim, Burton, & Lindsay, 1982). Perras and Zappacosta (1986) reported reduced peritonitis rates in CAPD from a combination of patient education and use of germicidal skin care.

Long-Term Education for Caregivers and Patients

Follow-up and retraining needs are important researchable problems for all areas of technological home care (Burton, Kline, Lindsay, & Heidenheim, 1988). Although follow-up visits are part of the federal Medicare policy for home dialysis reimbursement, the guidelines are vague. Effectiveness of follow-up home visits for 36 home peritoneal dialysis patients was evaluated by a nurse, a dietitian, and a social worker over an 18-month period (Ponferrada et al., 1993). This team made an average of four recommendations per home visit on the basis of family interactions, degree of independence and self-care, use of community resources, infection control, sexuality, and other new information gained. The recommendations were that a team or a community-health professional in consultation with a team should make home visits with structured guidelines for assessments. In a study of outcomes of instruction to caregivers managing home external cardioversion on cardiopulmonary resuscitation (CPR) via telephone, researchers found significantly better performance when specific words were used to prompt recall of previous training (Carter, Eisenberg, Hallstrom, & Schaeffer, 1984). Teaching by telephone or other media in the home needs further study. Problem-solving ability has been suggested as an important component of the successful management of home technology; however, no studies were found in which techniques of problem solving were taught. Evaluating patient and caregiver knowledge and techniques for home care periodically is an important area that deserves further study.

Caregiving Education for Support at Home

Needs for caregiver support groups were mentioned in most care plans or teaching protocols. However, this recommendation may be unrealistic for homebound caregivers if the patient cannot be left alone (Payne-James & Ball, 1991). Caregivers perceive visits from friends as important but report some visits as intrusive or poorly timed in the illness sequence, and many feel obligated to clean house, serve refreshments, or reciprocate the assistance. The use of computer networks is a method for linking homebound patients and providing a network or support group. Brennan, Moore, and Smyth (1991) reported on a randomized field study of a computer network linking caregivers of the elderly. The network facilitated communication, information exchange, and decision-making support between caregivers and nurses (Brennan, Moore, & Smyth, 1995).

Zahr and Montijo (1993) reported an evaluation study of a home care delivery program that provided service for family caregivers of low birth weight infants requiring phototherapy, intravenous therapy, mechanical ventilation, and apnea monitors. The home care program included 8 to 24 hours per day of nursing care and discharge education that included information about families' rights and responsibilities and about services that home nursing care would provide. This program used evaluation visits to the home prior to and 72 hours after the infant's discharge. Monthly nursing conferences and bimonthly updates of the medical plan also were used. In the 40 infants studied, the rehospitalization rate, mean number of emergency room visits, and doctor's office visits were less than those reported in previous studies for low birth weight infants. No data on family satisfaction were reported. Clinical models of comprehensive interventions or family-centered approaches for delivering technological home care services might also be fruitful in guiding research (Brooten et al., 1988; Ingersoll, Hoffart, & Schultz, 1990; Kaufman & Hardy-Ribakow, 1987; Saba, O'Hare, Boondas, Levine, & Oatway, 1992).

COSTS OF CAREGIVING WITH HOME CARE TECHNOLOGIES

Caregiving costs include direct financial expenditures, indirect costs in loss of employment, and psychosocial drain. Direct costs of home care are substantially less than institutional care. Costs were saved by third-party payors, not by family caregivers (C. E. Smith, 1995). Several researchers have indicated that costs relate to caregiving characteristics such as age, hours per day of care, and years of caring and that the relationship between the patient and caregiver predicts resources used and outcomes of care (Albrecht, 1991; Biegel, Sales, & Schulz, 1991; Given et al., 1992; Montgomery, Goneyea, & Hooymen, 1985; Wegener & Aday, 1989). Albrecht (1991) psychometrically established the reliability and validity of an instrument for workload analysis of home care nurses to predict nursing visits, based on severity of client problems; physical, psychosocial, and teaching needs; difficulty of the clinical judgment needed; and multiagency involvement.

The Brunier and McKeever (1993) review of 48 studies on the impact of home dialysis on families identified how caregivers frequently took on all aspects of care and then reported strain, anxiety, fatigue, and deteriorating relations with the patients. Caregivers' health succumbs to disruptive schedules and fatigue, which generate more health care bills. Challenges caregivers face include the stress of learning to manage the technology, few resources, and difficulty of accepting help from others (Corby, Schad, & Fudge, 1986; Davis, 1980; Miller, 1985; C. E. Smith, Moushey, Marien, & Weber, 1993). Caregivers perceive that they become socially isolated after friends stop visiting, but they also worry about their inability to return favors to friends (Payne-James & Ball, 1991). Overall, these studies depict caregiver stressors as the demanding physical care of the patient, disruptive scheduling of treatment regimens, mobilization of help from extended family or friends, management of household and financial affairs, and at times, observation of the patient's worsening condition. Financial and relationship stability were also key factors influencing depression and strain experienced by caregivers. Caregivers describe limited social lives, loss of privacy in the home, disruption in sleep, difficult schedules, demanding physical care, and curtailed activities of other family members (Gipson et al., 1987; Goldberg, 1986; C. E. Smith, Mayer, et al., 1991). Successful caregiving was related to patients' and caregivers' abilities to share responsibility, clarify tasks, and communicate before deciding how to respond to technical concerns.

No reported research was found on testing interventions that support family caregivers of technologically dependent adults. There is a lack of empirical information about the contribution nursing care makes to quality of life in these families. The studies of parents of technologically dependent children have confirmed the fatigue and stress of everyday life, the decisions to have no other children, the economic strain, and the career or employment hindrance placed on these caregivers. However, only few studies compared interventions or alternatives in delivery of care (Lobosco et al., 1991; Wegener & Aday, 1989). Intervention research from other groups of caregivers whom patients depend on for home care probably should be replicated for technological home care to develop clinically relevant suggestions for care.

Limitations of caregiving intervention studies include no testing of efficiency of the intervention prior to use, no attention paid to the timing of the intervention in the stage of caregiving, short-term measures of outcomes, few controlled comparison group studies, and no examination of differential effects of the intervention by gender or other pertinent caregiver variables (age, hours of care). Studies are needed that determine what parts of a multifaceted intervention enhance effects for the patient, caregiver, and family members. Brunier and McKeever (1993) point out that a theoretical basis has not been used in research of technological home care, and the conceptual links between family coping and stressors have not been verified in relationship to gender, economic, or societal issues.

CONCLUSIONS AND FUTURE RESEARCH DIRECTIONS

Synthesis of study findings from this review reveals that technologically dependent patients do perceive that they have quality in their lives related to improvement in their physical status. Acceptable quality of life from the techno-logically dependent patients' and caregivers' points of view has been verified although measured only superficially. Studies of individuals' experiences of tech-nological dependency, or how it feels to be connected to a machine, are needed (Gries & Fernsler, 1988; O'Brien, 1983; Schmeck, 1965). Home care was rated by patients and family members as more acceptable than institutionalization.

Generally, it is acknowledged that costs were saved over hospital care but then shifted to families who provided home nursing care. Ample data document the economic and emotional strain resulting from reimbursement regulations and from loss of income due to hindrance for both patients and caregivers. Attempts at comparing families' uses of their own caregiving resources and conserving their own health care benefits (federal or private) is an important area of research for the future. Also, analysis of cost-benefit outcomes related to the type of service delivery systems used is needed (Goldberg, 1983). The payment and quality assurance mechanisms are shaping the future of technology health care in the 1990s and beyond (DeLissovoy & Feustle, 1991).

Even though caregivers described limited social lives, loss of privacy in the home, disruption in sleep, difficult schedules, demanding physical care, and curtailed activities of other family members, the vast majority want the patient at home. Families described patient education at hospital discharge as providing them with confidence and the skills they needed to manage the machines and sterilization equipment. However, family members experienced anxiety related to learning the complicated technological care and transfer-ring it into the home setting (Schneider & Mirtallo, 1981). These problems have been reported to recur depending on the patient's condition and factors such as disease exacerbation, the ability to return to work, and availability of family support or external resources (C. E. Smith, Fernengel, Werkowitz, & Holcroft, 1992). Health professionals consistently confirm that an experienced multidisciplinary health care team is essential for assisting families in man-aging home technology. In contrast, the research reviewed herein documented that not all families had access to skilled teams. In fact, family members served as their own health care team. Thus, research studies must conceptualize fami-lies as systems of health care and delineate specific variables predictive of successful home care systems.

Reactions to home technology responsibilities have been addressed; however, extensive or longitudinal evaluations of caregiver effectiveness are limited (Lindeman, 1992). Another priority is to conduct studies with the family as the unit of analysis. The complexity of learning how to manage home technology has been investigated. Needs for retraining patients and caregivers are still unknown. Future studies evaluating media-based teaching should be based on a patient education framework (Lindeman, 1988, 1989).

Reactions of families to home technology have been addressed superficially by comparing this choice to a preference for institutionalization. However, more sensitive evaluations of social isolation, family dysfunction, and long-term impacts of home care are needed. Evaluations of the mainstreaming of technologically dependent children into schools and adults into the workplace also are needed, as well as longitudinal research on caregivers' career disruptions and employment hindrances. Nurses could implement data-based interventions and appropriate patient education for managing home technology in partnership with family caregivers who manage care in the home.

This review revealed that only after a home care technology is well entrenched are studies addressing ethical issues, patient and caregiver education, or quality of life undertaken. Such issues should be a part of all future studies (Haddad, 1992; Hoffart, 1989) and should be discussed in nursing curricula (Hegyvary, 1993). Further research may uncover other ethical and philosophical issues, such as the families' rights versus obligations, or prolonging life when quality is diminished (R. C. Fox, 1981; R. C. Fox, Swazey, & Cameron, 1984; Glendinning, 1994; Mitcham, 1994; Narins, 1984; Postman, 1992; Reckling, 1989; Sikorski, 1993). Such findings will create a need for a policy analysis type of research (R. W. Evans, Blagg, & Bryan, 1981; Goldberg, 1986; Jacox, 1992; Jones, 1987; Plough & Berry, 1981; Schmidt, Blumenkrantz, & Wiegmann, 1983).

ACKNOWLEDGMENT

Roma Lee Taunton, PhD, RN, FAAN, is acknowledged for her ongoing encouragement and support. Thank you to colleagues for their helpful comments. Jennifer Prather's manuscript preparation is greatly appreciated.

REFERENCES

Albrecht, M. N. (1991). Home health care: Reliability and validity testing of a patient-classification instrument. *Public Health Nursing, 8*, 124–131.

Alexander, S. R., Lindblad, A. S., Nolph, K. D., & Novak, J. W. (1990). Pediatric CAPD/CCPD in the United States. In J. H. Stein (Ed.), *Peritoneal dialysis* (pp. 231–255). New York: Churchill Livingstone.

American College of Physicians. (1989). Parenteral nutrition in patients receiving cancer chemotherapy. *Annals of Internal Medicine, 110,* 734–735.

Andre, J. (1986). Home health care and high-tech medical equipment. *Caring, 5*(9) 9–12.

Arras, J. D. (1994). The technological tether: An introduction to ethical and social issues in high-tech home care [Special supplement]. *Hastings Center Report, 24*(5), 51–52.

Atcherson, E., & Lowry, M. R. (1981). Home hemodialysis training: Factors affecting mastery. *American Association of Nephrology Nurses and Technicians Journal, 8,* 21–23.

Barnard, K., Hammond, M., Sumner, G. A., Kang, R., Johnson-Crowley, N., Snyder, C., Spietz, A., Blackburn, S., Brandt, P., & Magyary, D. (1987). Helping parents with preterm infants: Field test of a protocol. *Early Child Development and Care, 27,* 255–290.

Bayer, R. (1987). Ethical challenges: What does social justice demand in the provision of home health services? *Generations,11*(2), 44–46.

Benner, P. (1985). Quality of life: A phenomenological perspective on explanation, prediction, and understanding in nursing science. *Advances in Nursing Science, 8*(l), 1–14.

Bergstrom, N. (1986). Selecting methods to measure nutrition outcomes. *Oncology Nursing Forum, 13*(1), 96–98.

Biegel, D. E., Sales, E., & Schulz, R. (1991). *Family caregiving in chronic illness.* Newbury Park, CA: Sage.

Bihl, M. A., Ferrans, C. E., & Powers, M. J. (1988). Comparing stressors and quality of life of dialysis patients. *American Nephrology Nurses Association Journal, 15,* 27–37.

Boutin, J., & Hagan, E. (1992). Patients' preference regarding portable pumps. *Journal of Intravenous Nursing, 15,* 230–232.

Brennan, P. F., Moore, S. M., & Smyth, K. A. (1991). Computerlink: Electronic support for the home caregiver. *Advances in Nursing Science, 13*(4), 14–27.

Brennan, P. F., Moore, S. M., & Smyth, K. A. (1995). The effects of a special computer network on caregivers of persons with Alzheimer's disease. *Nursing Research, 44,* 166–171.

Brooten, D., Brown, L. P., Hazard-Munro, B., York, R., Cohen, S. M., Roncoli, M., & Hollingsworth, A. (1988). Early discharge and specialist transitional care. *Image: Journal of Nursing Scholarship, 20,* 64–68.

Brunier, G. M., & McKeever, P. T. (1993). The impact of home dialysis on the family: Literature review. *American Nephrology Nurses Association Journal, 20,* 653–659.

Bryan, F. A., & Evans, R. W. (1980). Hemodialysis partners. *Kidney International, 17,* 350–356.

Burton, H. J., Kline, S. A., Lindsay, R. M., & Heidenheim, P. (1988). The role of support in influencing outcome of end-stage renal disease. *General Hospital Psychiatry, 10,* 260–266.

Carter, W. B., Eisenberg, M. S., Hallstrom, A. P., & Schaeffer, S. (1984). Development and implementation of emergency CPR instruction via telephone. *Annals of Emergeny Medicine, 13,* 695–700.

Copeman, E., & Weigel, L. (1987). Training homemaker-home health aides for high-tech home care. *Caring, 6(15),* 34–37.

Corby, D. Schad, R. F., & Fudge, J. P. (1986). Intravenous antibiotic therapy: Hospital to home. *Nursing Management, 17*(8), 52–61.

Daly, B. J., Newlon, B., Montenegro, H. D., & Langdon, T. (1993). Withdrawal of mechanical ventilation: Ethical principles and guidelines for terminal weaning. *American Journal of Critical Care, 2,* 217–223.

Davis, A. J. (1980). Disability, home care, and the care-taking role in family life. *Journal of Advanced Nursing, 5,* 475–484.

Dekeyser, F. G. (1990). *Psychosocial factors and peritoneal immune function in CAPD patients.* Baltimore: University of Maryland.

DeLissovoy, G., & Feustle, J. A. (1991). Advanced home health care. *Health Policy, 17*, 227–242.

Detsky, A. S., McLaughlin, J. R., Abrams, H. B., L'Abbe, K. A., Whitwell, J., Bombardier, C., & Jeejeebhoy, K. A. (1986). Quality of life of patients on long term total parenteral nutrition at home. *General Internal Medicine, 1*, 26.

Diehl, S. F., Moffitt, K. A., & Wade, S. M. (1991). Focus group interview with parents of children with medically complex needs: An intimate look at their perceptions and feelings. *Children's Health Care, 20*, 170–178.

Eschbach, J. W., Egrie, J. C., Downing, M. R., Browne, J. K., & Adamson, J. W. (1987). Correction of the anemia of end-stage renal disease with recombinant human erythropoietin: Results of a combined phase I and II clinical trial. *New England Journal of Medicine, 316*, 73–78.

Evans, J. H., Daly, P. V., Kobayashi, R. H. Kobayashi, A. D. (1988). Quality of life correlates and psychological effects of home-based intravenous IgG infusion therapy [Abstract]. *Journal of Allergy and Clinical Immunology, 81*, 288.

Evans, R. W., Blagg, C. R., & Bryan, F. A. (1981). Implications for health care policy: A social and demographic profile of hemodialysis patients in the United States. *Journal of the American Medical Association, 245*, 487–491.

Evans, R. W., Manninen, D., Garrison, L., Hart, C., Blagg, C., Gutman, M., Hull, M., & Lowrie, M. (1985). Quality of life of patients with endstage renal disease. *New England Journal of Medicine, 312*, 553–559.

Fishman, D. B., & Schneider, C. J. (1972). Predicting emotional adjustment in home dialysis patients and their relatives. *Journal of Chronic Diseases, 25*, 99–109.

Foundation for Hospice and Homecare. (1987, May). *Crisis of chronically ill children in America: Triumph of technology—failure in policy.* Paper presented to U.S. Congress, Washington, DC.

Fox, E., Peace, K., Neale, T. J., Morrison, R. B., Hatfield, P. J., & Mellsop, G. (1991). Quality of life for patients with end-stage renal failure. *Renal Failure, 13*(1), 31–35.

Fox, R. C. (1981). Exclusion from dialysis: A sociologic and legal perspective. *Kidney International, 19*, 739–751.

Fox, R. C., Swazey, J. P., & Cameron, E. M. (1984). Social and ethical problems in the treatment of end-stage renal disease patients. In R. G. Narins (Ed.), *Controversies in nephrology and hypertension* (pp. 45–70). New York: Churchill Livingstone.

Frace, R. M. (1986). Home ventilation: An alternative to institutionalization. *Focus on Critical Care, 13*(6), 28–34.

Frates, R. C., Splaingard, M. L., Smith, E. O., & Harrison, G. M. (1985). Outcome of home mechanical ventilation for children. *Journal of Pediatrics, 106*, 850–856.

Fry, S. T. (1990). Ethical issues in total parenteral nutrition. *Nutrition, 6*, 329–331.

Geary, P. A. (1989). Stress and social support in the experience of monitoring apneic infants. *Clinical Nurse Specialist, 3*, 119–125.

Gipson, W. T., Sivak, E. D., & Gulledge, A. D. (1987). Psychological aspects of ventilator dependency. *Psychiatric Medicine, 5*, 245–255.

Given, C. W., Given, B., Stommel, M., Collins, C., King, S., & Franklin, S. (1992). The Caregiver Reaction Assessment (CRA) for caregivers to persons with chronic physical and mental impairments. *Research in Nursing and Health, 15*, 271–283.

Glendinning, C. (1994). *When technology wounds: Human consequences of progress.* New York: William Morrow.

Goldberg, A. I. (1983). Home care for a better life for ventilator-dependent people. *Chest, 84,* 365.

Goldberg, A. I. (1986). Home care for life-supported persons: Is a national approach the answer? *Chest, 90,* 744–748.

Goldberg, A. I., Noah, Z. N., Fleming, N., Staniek, L., Childs, B., Frost, L., & Glynn, W. (1987). Quality of care for life-supported children who require prolonged mechanical ventilation at home. *Quality Review Bulletin, 13*(3), 81–88.

Goldstein, M. (1991). Patient learning center reduces patient readmissions. *Patient Education and Counseling, 17,* 177–190,

Gonsalves-Ebrahim, L., Sterin, G., Gulledge, A. D., Gipson, W. T., & Rodgers, D. A. (1987). Noncompliance in younger adults on hemodialysis. *Psychosomatics, 28,* 34–41.

Gries, M. L., & Fernsler, J. F. (1988). Patient perceptions of the mechanical ventilation experience. *Focus on Critical Care, 15,* 52–59.

Guilleminault, C., Quera-Salva, M. A., Partinen, M., & Jamieson, A. (1988). Women and the obstructive sleep apnea syndrome. *Chest, 93,* 104–109.

Gurklis, J. A., & Menke, E. M. (1988). Identification of stressors and use of coping methods in chronic hemodialysis patients. *Nursing Research, 37,* 236–239.

Haddad, A. M. (1992). Ethical problems in home healthcare. *Journal of Nursing Administration, 22*(3), 46–51.

Hart, G. L., & Evans, R. W. (1987). The functional status of ESRD patients as measured by the Sickness Impact Profile. *Journal of Chronic Diseases, 40,* 117S–130S.

Hatz, P. S., & Powers, M. J. (1980). Factors related to satisfaction with life for patients on hemodialysis. *American Association of Nephrology Nurses and Technicians Journal, 7,* 290–295.

Heaphy, L. (1988, November-December). Survey results provide insight into psychosocial issues. *Lifeline Letter of Oley Foundation,* pp. 1–2.

Hegyvary, S. T. (1993). *A vision for nursing education.* (Available from National League for Nursing, 350 Hudson Street, New York, NY 10014).

Herfindal, E. T., Bernstein, L. R., Kudzia, K., & Wong, A. (1989). Survey of home nutritional support patients. *Journal of Parenteral and and Enteral Nutrition, 13,* 255–261.

Hoffart, N. (1989). Nephrology nursing, 1915–1970: A historical study of the integration of technology and care. *American Nephrology Nurses' Association Journal, 16,* 169–178.

Howard, L. (1992). Home parenteral nutrition in patients with a cancer diagnosis. *Journal of Parenteral and Enteral Nutrition, 16,* 935–995.

Ingersoll, G. L., Hoffart, N., & Schultz, A. W. (1990). Health services research in nursing: Current status and future directions. *Nursing Economics, 8,* 229–238.

Institute of Medicine Staff. (1989). *Quality of life and technology assessment.* Washington, DC: National Academy Press.

Jacox, A. (1992). Health care technology and its assessment: Where nursing fits in. In L. Aiken & C. Fagin (Eds.), *Charting nursing's future: Agenda for the 1990's* (pp. 70–84). Philadelphia: Lippincott.

Jeffrey, J. E., Heidenheim, A. P., Burton, H. J., & Lindsay, R. M. (1982). A comparison of home training and problems encountered with initial home dialysis:

Hemodialysis vs. CAPD. *American Association of Nephrology Nurses and Technicians Journal, 9*, 56–62.

Jones, K. R. (1987). Policy and research in end-stage renal disease. *Image: Journal of Nursing Scholarship, 19*, 126–129.

Kaufman, J., & Hardy-Ribakow, D. (1987). Home care: A model of a comprehensive approach for technology-assisted chronically ill children. *Journal of Pediatric Nursing, 2*, 244–249.

King, F. E., Figge, J., & Jarman, P. (1986). The elderly coping at home: A study of continuity of nursing care. *Journal of Advanced Nursing, 11*, 41–46.

Klein, S., Simes, J., & Blackburn, G. L. (1986). Total parenteral nutrition and cancer clinical trials. *Cancer, 58*, 1378–1386.

Knox, L. S. (1989). Ethical issues in nutritional support. *Nursing Clinics of North America, 24*, 427–438.

Kruger, S., & Rawlins, P. (1984). Pediatric dismissal protocol to aid the transition from hospital care to home care. *Image: Journal of Nursing Scholarship, 16*, 120–125.

Kuhn, B. G. (1980). Prediction of nursing requirements from patients' characteristics: 2. *International Journal of Nursing Studies, 17*, 5–15.

Ladefoged, K. (1980). Quality of life in patients on permanent home parenteral nutrition. *Journal of Parenteral and Enteral Nutrition, 5*, 132–137.

Laine, L. L., Shulman, R. J., Gardner, P., Bartholomew, K., Reed, T., & Cole, S. (1988). An educational booklet can diminish anxiety in parents whose children receive total parenteral nutrition. *Journal of Parenteral and Enteral Nutrition, 12*, 11.

Lange, M. H. (1986). Managing Blue Cross and Blue Shield benefits for high-tech home care. *Caring, 5*(9), 58–60.

Lansky, D., Doerr, H. O., & Ivey, M. (1982). Teaching home parenteral nutrition to patients with limited compliance skills. *Journal of Parenteral and Enteral Nutrition, 6*, 160–162.

Lindeman, C. A. (1988). Patient education: Part 1. In J. J. Fitzpatrick, R. L. Taunton, & J. Q. Benoliel (Eds.), *Annual review of nursing research* (Vol. 6, pp. 19–60). New York: Springer Publishing Co.

Lindeman, C. A. (1989). Patient education: Part 2. In J. J. Fitzpatrick, R. L. Taunton, & J. Q. Benoliel (Eds.), *Annual review of nursing research* (Vol. 7, pp. 199–212). New York: Springer Publishing Co.

Lindeman, C. A. (1992). Nursing and technology: Moving into the 21st century. *Caring, 11*(9), 7–10.

Lindgren, C. (1987, May). *Stress, anxiety, burnout, and social support in family caregivers.* Paper presented at Sigma Theta Tau International, Edinburgh, Scotland.

Lobosco, A. F., Eron, N. B., Bobo, T., Kril, L., & Chalanick, K. (1991). Local coalitions for coordinating services to children dependent on technology and their families. *Children's Health Care, 20*, 75–86.

Lowry, M. R., & Atcherson, E. (1980). A short-term follow-up of patients with depressive disorder on entry into home dialysis training. *Journal of Affective Disorders, 2*, 219–227.

Mattox, T. W. (1993). Drug use evaluation approach to monitoring use of total parenteral nutrition: A review of criteria for use in cancer patients. *Nutrition in Clinical Practice, 8*, 233–237.

Miller, A. (1985). When is the time ripe for teaching? *American Journal of Nursing.* *85*, 801–804.

Millner, B. N. (1991). Technology-dependent children in New York State. *Bulletin of New York Academy of Medicine, 67,* 131–142.

Mitcham, C. (1994). *Thinking through technology: The path between engineering and philosophy.* Chicago: University of Chicago Press.

Molzahn, A. E. (1991). The reported quality of life of selected home hemodialysis patients. *American Nephrology Nurses Association Journal, 18,* 173–181.

Montgomery, R., Goneyea, J., & Hooyman, N. (1985). Caregiving and the experience of subjective and objective burden. *Family Relations, 34,* 19–26.

Motwani, J. K., & Herring, G. M. (1988). Home care for ventilator-dependent persons: A cost-effective, humane, public policy. *Health and Social Work, 13,* 20–24.

Narins, R. G. (Ed.). (1984). *Controversies in nephrology and hypertension.* Orlando, FL: Grune and Stratton.

National Academy of Sciences. (1995). *Workshop on human factors and home medical equipment* (Report of National Research Council and National Academy of Science, Committee on Human Factors.) Washington, DC: Author.

OLEY/A.S.P.E.N. Information System (OASIS) (1987–89). *Home nutrition support patient registry: Annual reports, 1985–1986, 1987.* Albany, NY: Oley Foundation.

O'Brien, M. E. (1983). *The courage to survive: The life career of the chronic dialysis patient.* New York: Grune & Stratton.

Palmer. S. E., Canzona, L., & Wai, L. (1982) Helping families respond effectively to chronic illness: Home dialysis as a case example. *Social Work in Health Care, 8,* 1–14.

Payne, S. A. (1992). A study of quality of life in cancer patients receiving palliative chemotherapy. *Social Sciences Medicine, 35,* 1505–1509.

Payne-James, J., & Ball, P. (1991). Support group for patients receiving home nutritional support. *British Journal of Hospital Medicine, 46,* 269.

Perras, S. T., & Zappacosta, A. R. (1986). Reduction of peritonitis with patient education and the Travenol CAPD Germicidal Exhange Device. *American Nephrology Nurses Association Journal, 13,* 219–222.

Peterson, K. J. (1985). Psychosocial adjustment of the family caregiver: Home hemodialysis as an example. *Social Work in Health Care, 10*(3), 15–33.

Plough, A. C., & Berry, R. E. (1981). Regulating medical uncertainty: Policy issues in end-stage renal disease. In Altman, D. & Sapolsky, H. M. (Eds.), *Federal health programs: Problems and prospects* (pp. 153–176). Lexington, MA: Heath.

Plummer, A. L., O'Donohue, W. J., & Petty, T. L. (1989). Consensus conference on problems in home mechanical ventilation. *American Review of Respiratory Disease, 140,* 555–560.

Ponferrada, L., Burrows, L. M., Prowant, B., Satalowich, R. J., Schmidt, L. M., & Bartelt, C. (1993). Home visit effectiveness for peritoneal dialysis patients. *American Nephrology Nurses Association Journal, 20,* 333–336.

Postman, N. (1992). *Technopoly: The surrender of culture to technology.* New York: Alfred A. Knopf.

Reckling, J. B. (1989). Abandonment of patients by home health nursing agencies: An ethical analysis of the dilemma. *Advances in Nursing Sciences, 11*(3), 70–81.

Rettig, R. A., & Levinsky, N. G. (Eds.). (1991). *Committee for the study of the Medicare ESRD program, Division of Health Care Services.* Washington, DC: National Academy Press.

Roberts, J. C., & Kjellstrand, C. M. (1988). Choosing death: Withdrawal from chronic dialysis without medical reason. *ACTA Medical Scandinavica, 223,* 181–186.

Roy, C., Flynn, E., & Atcherson, E. (1980). Home hemodialysis and the older patient. *American Association of Nephrology Nurses and Technicians Journal, 7,* 317–324.

Rydholm, L., & Pauling, J. (1991). Contrasting feelings of helplessness in peritoneal and hemodialysis patients: A pilot study. *American Nephrology Nurses Association Journal, 18,* 183–186.

Saba, V., O'Hare, P., Boondas, J., Levine, E., & Oatway, D. (1992). A nursing intervention taxonomy for home health care. *Nursing Scan in Research, 12,* 296–299.

Schmeck, H. M. (1965). *The semi-artificial man.* New York: Walker.

Schmidt, R. W., Blumenkrantz, M., & Wiegmann, T. B. (1983). The dilemmas of patient treatment for end-stage renal disease. *American Journal of Kidney Disease, 3,* 37–47.

Schneider. P. J., & Mirtallo, J. M. (1981). Home parenteral nutrition programs. *Journal of Parenteral and Enteral Nutrition, 5,* 157–160.

Sikorski, W. (1993). *Modernity and technology.* Tuscaloosa: University of Alabama Press.

Simmons, R. G. & Abress, L. (1990). Quality-of-life issues for end-stage renal disease patients. *American Journal of Kidney Diseases, 15,* 201–208.

Simmons, R. G., Anderson, C. R., & Kamstra, L. K. (1984). Comparison of quality of life of patients on CAPD, hemodialysis and transplantation, *American Journal of Kidney Diseases, 4,* 253–255.

Singer, P., Rothkopf, M. M., Kvetan, V., Kirvela, O., Gaare, J., & Askanazi, J. (1991). Risks and benefits of home parenteral nutrition in the acquired immunodeficiency syndrome. *Journal of Parenteral and Enteral Nutrition. 15,* 75–79.

Smith, C. E. (1993). Quality of life in long-term total parenteral nutrition patients and their family caregiver. *Journal of Parenteral and Enteral Nutrition, 17,* 501–506.

Smith, C. E. (1995). Technology and home care. In J. J. Fitzpatrick & J. S. Stevenson (Eds.) *Annual review of nursing research* (Vol. 13, pp. 137–167). New York: Springer Publishing Co.

Smith, C. E., Faust-Wilson, P., Lohr, G., Kallenberger, S., & Marien, L. (1992). A measure of distress reaction to diarrhea in ventilated tube-fed patients. *Nursing Research, 41,* 312–313.

Smith, C. E., Fernengel, K., Werkowitz, M., & Holcroft, C. (1992). Financial and psychological costs of high technology home care. *Nursing Economics, 10,* 369–372.

Smith, C. E., Giefer, C. K., & Bieker, L. (1991). Technological dependency: A preliminary model and pilot of home total parenteral nutrition. *Journal of Community Health Nursing, 8,* 245–254.

Smith, C. E., Mayer, L., Parkhurst, C., Perkins, S., & Pingleton, S. (1991). Adaptation in families with a member requiring mechanical ventilation at home. *Heart and Lung, 20,* 349–356.

Smith, C. E., Mayer, L. S., Perkins, S. B., Gerald, K., & Pingleton, S. K. (1994). Caregiver learning needs and reactions to managing home mechanical ventilation. *Heart and Lung, 23,* 157–163.

Smith, C. E., Moushey, L. M., Marien, L., & Weber, P. (1993). Family caregiver's perceptions of important knowledge and skills needs for managing total parenteral nutrition in the home. *Journal of Patient Education and Counseling, 21,* 155–164.

Smith, C. E., Moushey, L. M., Ross, J. A., & Giefer, C. (1993). Responsibilities and reactions of family caregivers of patients dependent on total parenteral nutrition at home. *Public Health Nursing, 10,* 122–128.

Smith, M., Hang, B. A., Michelman, J. E., & Robson, A. M. (1983). Treatment bias in the management of end-stage renal disease. *American Journal of Kidney Diseases, 3,* 21–26.

Soskolne, V., & DeNour, A. K. (1987). Psychosocial adjustment of home hemodialysis, continuous ambulatory peritoneal dialysis and hospital dialysis patients and their spouses. *Nephronology, 47,* 266–273.

Splaingard, M. L., Frates, R. C., Jr., Harrison, G. M., Carter, R. I., & Jefferson, L. S. (1983). Home positive-pressure ventilation: Twenty years' experience. *Chest, 84,* 376–382.

Srivastava, R. H. (1988). Coping strategies used by spouses of CAPD patients. *American Nephrology Nurses Association Journal, 15,* 174–179.

Steele, N., & Harrison, B. (1986). Technology-assisted children: Assessing discharge preparation. *Journal of Pediatric Nursing, 1,* 150–158.

Stiller, S. B. (1988). Success and difficulty in high-tech home care. *Public Health Nursing, 5,* 68–75.

Sweeney, L. B. (1988). Impact on families caring for an infant with apnea. *Issues in Comprehensive Pediatric Nursing, 11,* 1–15.

Thomas, V. M., Ellison, K., Howell, E. V., & Winters, K. (1992). Caring for the person receiving ventilatory support at home: Care givers' needs and involvement. *Heart and Lung, 21,* 180–186.

Thompson, C. L., & Richmond, M. (1990). Teaching home care for ventilator-dependent patients: The patients' perception. *Heart and Lung, 19,* 79–83.

Torrance, G. W. (1987). Utility approach to measuring health-related quality of life. *Journal of Chronic Diseases, 40,* 593–603.

Torrance, G. W., Boyle, M. H., & Horwood, S. P. (1982). Application of multiattribute utility theory to measure social preferences for health states. *Operations Research, 30,* 1043–1069.

U.S. Congress, Office of Technology Assessment. (1987a). Mechanical ventilation. In *Life sustaining technology and the elderly* (OTA-BA-306). Washington, DC: U.S. Government Printing Office.

U.S. Congress, Office of Technology Assessment, Health Program. (1987b). Technology-dependent children: Hospital vs. home care—a technical memorandum (OTA-TM-H-38). Washington, DC: U.S. Government Printing Office.

Wegener, D. H., & Aday, L. A. (1989). Home care for ventilator-assisted children: Predicting family stress. *Pediatric Nursing, 15,* 371–376.

Weinstein, M. C. (1983). Economic assessments of medical practices and technologies. *Medical Decision Making, 1,* 309–330.

Winearls, C. G., Oliver, D. O., Pippard, M. J., Reid, C., Downing, M. R., & Cotes, P. M. (1986). Effect of human erythropoietin derived from recombinant DNA on the anaemia of patients maintained by chronic haemodialysis. *Lancet, 2,* 1175–1178.

Zahr, L. K., & Montijo, J. (1993). The benefits of home care for sick premature infants. *Neonatal Network, 12*(1), 33–37.

PART II

Research on Nursing Care Delivery

Chapter 6

Organizational Redesign: Effect on Institutional and Consumer Outcomes

GAIL L. INGERSOLL
INDIANA UNIVERSITY SCHOOL OF NURSING

CONTENTS

Organizational redesign is most noticeable in hospitals, where innovative models are being developed to move the organizations from a product-focused to a market-focused orientation (Shortell, Morrison, & Friedman, 1992). Hospitals are introducing a variety of care-delivery models, most of which concentrate resources around patients with similar needs. Developers of the models have reported reductions in costs of staffing (Jones & Bullard, 1993) and in time spent in duplication of services (Cassidy, 1992). These reports are anecdotal, however, and few studies of their long-term effects have been conducted.

To determine the state of the science concerning the effect of organizational redesign on institutional and consumer outcomes, a comprehensive review of published literature was conducted for the years 1985 through 1994. For purposes of the review, *consumer* was defined as health care worker, patient, family, or member of the community. Health care workers are included because they constitute internal consumers of the organization, whereas patients, families, and community members constitute external consumers of services.

Studies were restricted to those in which researchers evaluated the effect of organizational redesign in hospitals and health care agencies. Community health initiatives were included if they incorporated identifiable organizations into the program. Reports of redesign projects in which no evaluation data were presented or where the findings were described in global terms were excluded from the review. Also excluded were reports of single-purpose care delivery interventions, such as those associated with delivery of home care services by nurses (e.g., Vines & Williams-Burgess, 1994), nurse extenders (e.g., Bray & Edwards, 1994), or agencies (e.g., McCorkle et al., 1994) and use of discharge planners (e.g., Mamon et al., 1992), case managers (e.g., Fleishman, Mor, & Piette, 1991), and advanced practice nurses (e.g., Brooten et al., 1986). The focus was restricted to studies of how changes in the care delivery structures of organizations affected institutional and consumer outcomes.

METHODS

Three methods were used to identify studies for review. A comprehensive computer search was conducted using nursing (Cumulative Index of Nursing and Allied Health Literature [CINAHL]), medical (MEDLINE), business (Business Index), and general academic topics indexes (CARL Uncover; Expanded Academic Index). Keywords used in the search included change, evaluation, health maintenance organization, innovation, model, outcome, redesign, and reorganization. In addition, individual issues for the years 1990 through 1994 were reviewed for journals most likely to publish reports of organizational redesign evaluations. These included *Academy of Management Journal, Advances in Nursing Science, Health Care Financing Review, Health Care Management Review, Health Services Research, Hospital and Health Services Administration, International Journal of Health Services* (1992–1994), *Journal of Healthcare Quality, Journal of Nursing Administration, Journal of Nursing Care Quality, Nursing Economics, Nursing Research,* and *Western Journal of Nursing Research.* Citations within research reports also were tracked for identification of other studies.

Studies reviewed were grouped according to extent of redesign initiative. Studies of first-order redesign were defined as those in which the overall organization remained unchanged while efforts were made to change subsystems within the institution (Meyer, Goes, & Brooks, 1993). Second-order redesigns were defined as those in which the fundamental properties or states of the organization changed. A third category (third-order redesign) was added for this review; it includes redesigns involving multiple organizations or community agencies.

These categories of redesign were used in the review because some individuals have reported that first-order (or bottom-up) redesigns are unlikely to produce any lasting effect on the organization (Dienemann & Gessner, 1992). They believe that the absence of involvement by influential persons within the organization makes these initiatives less likely to result in measurable outcomes. Studies to substantiate this perspective are lacking, however, and several reports have suggested that as long as there is support from senior management, measurable effect is possible (Cassard, Weisman, Gordon, & Wong, 1994; Zelauskas & Howes, 1992).

FINDINGS

Twenty-seven organizational redesign evaluation reports met the review's inclusion criteria and are described in this analysis. Of that number, 13 (48.2%) fell into the first-order redesign category, 8 (29.6%) into the second-order category, and 6 (22.2%) into the third. Four of the reports in the first category pertained to one study of a professional practice model introduced at Johns Hopkins Hospital. Two studies in the second-order category were described in two articles each, and one study in the third-order category was described in four. Consequently, the overall number of redesign evaluations reviewed for this analysis was 19, of which first-order redesigns outnumbered second- and third-order redesigns combined by 2 to 1.

Studies of First-Order Redesign

The 10 studies of first-order redesign examined the following models: modified primary nursing (Teresi et al., 1992); nurse extender (Garfink, Kirby, Bachman, & Starck, 1991); modified differentiated nursing practice (Malloch, Milton, & Jobes, 1990); decentralized decision making (Barhyte, Counte, & Christman, 1987); unit-based governance (Zelauskas & Howes, 1992); primary, team, or total patient care nursing (Clark & Zornow, 1989); feedback system (James, Milne, & Firth, 1990); professionally advanced care team (Brett & Tonges, 1990); psychiatric services (Hunter, Buick, Wellington, Dzerovych, 1993); and contract (Dear, Weisman, & O'Keefe, 1985). A primary concern about the overall impact of these studies is the variable time frame used for determination of effect. Evaluations occurred anywhere from 3 (Barhyte et al., 1987) to 30 months (Zelauskas & Howes, 1992), making comparisons across studies and assessment of true long-term effect difficult.

In the modified primary nursing model Teresi et al. (1992) evaluated the assignment of nursing attendants to provision of primary care in two long-term care facilities. They used a quasi-experimental matched group design to measure the effect of the model on staff morale and attitude toward primary nursing, staff and resident attitude toward permanent assignment of nursing attendants, and resident satisfaction with care. The two sites selected were a large institution with two special care units (one experimental and one comparison) and three nonspecial care units (two experimental and one comparison) and a small institution composed of one experimental and one comparison unit.

Staff and patient respondents completed questionnaires designed by the investigators. Instrument reliability was assessed through internal consistency procedures only. Cronbach's alpha ranged from .18 (resident attitude toward primary care at Time 2) to .89 (staff attitude toward primary care at Time 2) (Teresi et al., 1992). Low internal consistency estimates for the residents suggest that they had limited understanding of the construct measured. These findings also suggest that data for the scales were unreliable and unacceptable for analysis purposes.

Following implementation of the modified primary care model, experimental unit staff were more positive about their perceptions of permanent assignment for attendants. Negative perceptions were expressed concerning heaviness of work load and the need for long-term care of residents with behavior problems. At the larger facility, differences were seen in resident perceptions of overall satisfaction with care and attitudes toward primary care. No differences were seen for the smaller institution, where scale reliabilities were suspect and the total number of participants was small.

A qualitative component of this study was described in insufficient detail to merit review, although one comment noted by the authors reinforces the problems inherent in reporting evaluation findings at short intervals post-redesign initiative. One year after the modified primary care model was introduced, one institution had reverted to bimonthly rotation for attendants. The limited number of staff available to adjust assignments and the increased number of behaviorally disturbed residents necessitated the elimination of permanent assignment. Although troubling, this information is relevant and necessary for understanding the true long-term outcome of the redesign initiative.

In the nurse extender evaluation, data were collected 1 year after redesign implementation (Garfink et al., 1991). In this model, a registered nurse (RN) and patient care technician worked together to care for a group of patients. The evaluation of this first-order redesign consisted of a process component and an outcome component, which included an assessment of the model's impact on nurses' job satisfaction and patient care costs. An existing instrument was used to compare the job satisfaction of nurses on three redesigned units to the job satisfaction of nurses on three control units.

Cost of care was compared to the traditional primary care model in place at the study hospital. Actual hours of direct patient care per patient day, total patient days, and budgeted hours of direct patient care were measured for comparable periods. In addition, average actual hours per patient day and average weighted hourly salaries for care providers were calculated.

No differences in level of nurse satisfaction were seen between nurse extender and primary care units. Differences were seen between nurse extender and primary care units for average hourly wage, however. This reduction was the result of the use of less costly care providers and the reduction in number of RNs required to deliver care. The number of direct care delivery hours also declined.

The introduction of a modified differentiated practice model was evaluated by Malloch et al. (1990) at a community hospital in the Southwest. In this study, RN positions were differentiated by educational preparation into case manager (baccalaureate) and case associate (associate degree) roles. In addition, a unit assistant role was added, although how this individual fits within the differentiated model was less clearly defined. The intent of the role was to reduce the time case managers and case associates spent on nonnursing activities.

Effect of the model was measured on nurse satisfaction and patient and fiscal outcomes. In the report of findings, several problems were noted. First, no data were provided to substantiate the statement that nurses' satisfaction with task requirements and time to do the job increased significantly over time. More information was provided about vacancies on study units, although the time frame for reporting was somewhat uncertain. Second, the authors reported that evaluation data were collected prior to and at periodic intervals after the project was implemented, but no indication of the timing of intervals was provided.

Fiscal outcomes in this study were reported according to use of supplemental agency staff and worked hours per patient day, which were reduced following introduction of the model. How the introduction of a unit assistant, which was mentioned briefly in the report, contributed to the cost reduction was unclear. Consequently, whether the cost savings were the result of the differentiated practice model or the addition of the unit assistant is uncertain. Because overtime and worked hours per patient day may have been affected by the addition of the unit assistant, this was a serious limitation of the calculation of cost. Information about how this role was factored into the calculation would have been useful.

Patient outcomes were reported through counts of patient incidents per year. Both units involved in the project reported reductions in frequency of overall incidents and in falls and medication or intravenous errors. The authors noted that the actual number of incidents was small, however, so the magnitude of the effect was limited (Malloch et al., 1990). No information about sustained effect was provided.

In the Barhyte et al. (1987) study, decentralization of decision-making responsibility at the unit level was assessed in a large hospital located in the Midwest. Four nursing units in which a decentralized administrative approach was used were compared to four units in which a more bureaucratic approach was used by the nurse leader. Data pertaining to characteristics of the nurse, the unit, and job attendance behaviors were collected from staff nurses working on the units 1 month before the decentralized model was introduced and 3 and 6 months after model implementation. Semistructured interviews of unit leaders were conducted at the same time.

Decentralization was found to be an inverse predictor of leave taking, although leave taking was more strongly associated with previous leave-taking behavior. As a result, the researchers reported that the effect of decentralization on job attendance behavior was sporadic and uncertain (Barhyte et al., 1987).

Zelauskas and Howe (1992) used a quasi-experimental matched group design to measure the effect of a unit-based governance system on job characteristics, job satisfaction, recruitment and retention of nurses, quality assurance performance, unit cost per patient day, and utilization costs. In this redesign initiative, a decentralized decision-making process was introduced onto a 26-bed detoxification unit. Decision-making authority was granted through a committee structure created for purposes of overseeing unit and personnel management. Exempt salary status for employees was incorporated into the model.

Data pertaining to job satisfaction and job characteristics were collected at 6, 12, and 30 months after redesign implementation. Preimplementation data were available for staff job satisfaction only. Data on turnover, sick time, and cost per patient day were collected at baseline and at 12 and 30 months post-implementation (Zelauskas & Howes, 1992). This redesign evaluation is one of the few that reported data for more than one period after model implementation.

Differences were seen between experimental and comparison units for nursing education and experience, with experimental unit nurses being more experienced and more likely to be baccalaureate-prepared. No information was provided about how these differences may have contributed to study findings. Perceptions about the job in general and satisfaction with pay were rated more positively by experimental unit nurses at 6 months. Promotional opportunities were perceived more favorably by experimental units at 30 months (Zelauskas & Howes, 1992). All other variables were nonsignificant for differences.

Cost of the model was reported in percentage of change over time. A decline in cost occurred on the experimental unit despite salary increments for the all-RN staff and a mixed staffing pattern on the comparison unit. Nonsalary costs declined somewhat on both experimental and comparison units. Turnover rates declined for both units, although experimental unit declines were greater than for comparison unit or hospital.

Findings of this study reinforce the need to collect outcome data at more than one time. Differences seen at one data collection point disappeared by the time of the next one. Some differences were seen only at the last data collection. Had the researchers collected data only once, the true effect of the redesign might have been misrepresented.

In a study of nursing organizing systems (primary, team, or total patient care), investigators examined how efficient the models were for delivering patient care in a medium-sized community hospital (Clark & Zornow, 1989). Efficiency was defined as "the relative time spent in those nursing activities that involve direct care" (p. 759).

Researchers observed nursing personnel for a period of 6 weeks and categorized the types of activities seen during 30-minute sampling frames. Observations were made by the investigators during every hour of a 24-hour period and for every day of the week for each of the study units involved.

A total of 1,208 activities were observed during 236 observation periods. Of the activities observed on each of the units (two primary nursing, two team nursing, and four total patient care nursing), the most time was spent in direct care activities, although these accounted for only 19% of the time spent by nurses. Giving physical care (17%), observing patients (15%), and writing (14%) constituted the three most frequently observed tasks. No differences in efficiency of care were seen for the three types of organizing systems. This finding is clinically significant in light of the current tendency to reintroduce team nursing into primary nursing environments.

In a brief description of a feedback system for sharing information about special care unit atmosphere, James, Milne, and Firth (1990) reported on the effect of feedback on perception of unit atmosphere. Feedback in this study was provided either in written form alone or in written form in combination with opportunity for discussion. Although significant findings were reported for perception of work environment between groups, the number of participants in the study was small, the information provided about the study design and methods of analyses was limited, and the time frame for data collection was short (6 months). Consequently, this study represents one of the common problems observed in reports of research concerning organizational redesign: insufficient information to allow for careful critique of findings and failure to include discussion of potential limitations in study design and methods.

Brett and Tonges (1990) reported on an evaluation of a first-order redesign introduced at Robert Wood Johnson University Hospital. In this study of a professionally advanced care team (ProACT) model, a pre- and postintervention design was used to measure the effect of the model at 3 and 8 months postimplementation on a 32-bed surgical orthopedic unit. Information about timing of preintervention data collection was imprecise but apparently occurred immediately prior to the model's implementation.

The authors of this study described an evaluation plan designed to measure the extent of the "achievement of the model's objectives" (Brett & Tonges, 1990, p. 38), which were defined as (a) implementing a model that enables fewer RNs to provide care, (b) expanding clinical and nonclinical services at the unit level to free RNs for work only they can do, (c) maintaining primary nursing as the core of the nursing care delivery model, and (d) creating an expanded nursing role. Indicators of model effect were defined as patient satisfaction, job satisfaction, quality of nursing care, and cost of care delivery (Brett & Tonges, 1990). Although these outcome variables were reasonable and appropriate indicators of the effect of the model on internal and external consumers, they do not measure whether the model's objectives were achieved as stated.

Nonetheless, no differences in patient satisfaction scores were seen between baseline and 3 and 8 months postintervention. No differences in nurse satisfaction scores were seen either. Among the reasons for lack of findings in the patient sample may be the limited number of subjects; but because no information was provided about the sample size for the nursing staff, no assessment can be made about whether the number of subjects involved was sufficient to detect differences in perceptions.

Patient length of stay was reduced between baseline and 3 and 8 months after model implementation. Incidents per patient day remained constant, suggesting that reduction in RNs on the unit did not result in reduced quality of care. Unfortunately, the number of RNs reduced in the model is unknown; consequently, the helpfulness of these findings in terms of recent changes occurring in similar RN reduction models is limited.

Hunter, Buick, Wellington, and Dzerovych (1993) reported on a first-order study in which two locked inpatient units of a community mental health center's inpatient services were redesigned to provide acute-treatment day services, psychiatric intensive care, and transitional residence. The redesign they introduced was adapted from a second-order redesign project described below (Dickey et al., 1989; Gudeman, Dickey, Evans, & Shore, 1985). Effectiveness of the redesign was measured according to functional status of a 10% random sample of patients treated prior to and following introduction of the new program.

Two 10-month periods were compared, using data collected from the center's computerized information system and medical records. Level of functioning was determined by behavior/functioning status and frequency of episodes of seclusion and restraint. Findings showed that status level on day of discharge or transfer increased significantly after the redesign was initiated. The number of episodes of restraint use increased significantly also, although a decline was seen during the last month of data collection. The initial rise in restraint use was believed to be related to the increased number of admissions with complex, serious illnesses. The number of episodes of seclusion were comparable pre- and postredesign. When duration of stay was considered, however, use of seclusion as a treatment intervention declined significantly.

One of the more widely reported studies of first-order redesign is the Contract Model (Dear et al., 1985), later referred to as the Unit-Based Professional Practice Model (PPM) (Cassard et al., 1994; Weisman, Gordon, Cassard, Bergner, & Wong, 1993; Wong, Gordon, Cassard, Weisman, & Bergner, 1993) implemented at the Johns Hopkins Hospital. This model was introduced into one unit of the hospital and was then extended to 15 additional units, resulting in over one quarter of all hospital nursing units being included in the redesign process (Cassard et al., 1994).

To assess for the effect of the model on nurses' perceptions of work process, work satisfaction, and retention, Weisman et al. (1993) compared survey responses of nurses employed on 8 PPM units to 8 units matched for size and mix. They also monitored retention rates at 12 months postsurvey. Instruments used to measure job satisfaction and work process were modified or developed by the researchers; internal consistency reliability estimates were acceptable.

PPM nurses' perceptions of participation in decision making were significantly higher than those of comparison unit nurses. Overall work satisfaction also was significantly higher, with primary effect occurring through two work process variables: degree of care coordination and effectiveness of team performance. Nurse retention was unaffected by the model. Amount of pay, hours worked, and work satisfaction were predictive of retention.

The model's effect on patients was measured on four adult PPM nursing units that were matched to non-PPM units (Cassard et al., 1994). Subjects in the study were all patients admitted to units during a 3-month period in 1990. Of the 1,099 eligible patients seen during this period, 30% were enrolled in the study and were assessed on day of discharge for satisfaction with hospital and nursing care delivery. No differences were seen between units.

Two weeks postdischarge, subjects were contacted concerning patient outcome, which was defined as perceived health and functional status, met and unmet needs of care, and additional use of health care services, including readmission within 31 days of discharge. No differences were seen for perceived health and functional status or for additional health care utilization. Differences were seen, however, for met and unmet needs, with PPM patients reporting significantly more treatment-related needs, instrumental activities of daily living

(IADL) needs, and unmet IADL needs. When patient characteristics (e.g., age, sex, severity of illness, and length of stay) were controlled for in further analyses, however, the differences disappeared. Overall, no effect was seen for the PPM.

The cost of the model was assessed by comparing admission, patient days, and average length of stay data to productive and total hours worked by nursing staff. Cost expenditure data included salary and benefit figures plus unit expenditures on supplies, repairs, and services. One-year data were compared for eight experimental and eight comparison units (Wong et al., 1993). Findings showed the PPM units had higher patient loads, although the differences were not significant. Number of hours worked for aides and float pool nurses was significantly higher for inpatient non-PPM units. Number of RN hours worked was significantly higher for PPM specialty units (operating rooms). Overall, differences in cost were seen only for the PPM operating rooms, for which costs were significantly higher.

Studies of Second-Order Redesign

Reports of second-order redesign were fewer in number; although when reported, they were more complete in terms of description of design, methods, and analysis of findings. In one early report of a second-order evaluation of a nursing care partnerships (NCP) model, Schroeder and Maeve (1992) used a qualitative approach to collect data pertaining to the effect of the model on staff and clients. Because this model was introduced throughout an outpatient center designed to provide services for persons needing primary HIV/AIDS care, it is designated as second-order.

To determine nurse perceptions about strengths and weaknesses of the program, focus groups were conducted by the investigators (Schroeder & Maeve, 1992). Unfortunately, no information was provided about when these groups met. Moreover, the description of the findings was limited, and no discussion of methods used to analyze data was included.

To assess the effect of the model on nurse documentation, the authors reviewed medical records "several months" after the program was implemented. The medical record review assessed for evidence of inclusion of "carative" factors (caring activities) and the use of present and future focus in documentation. Twenty records were reviewed, of which 40% contained documentation concerning carative factors; less than half contained both a present and future focus (Schroeder & Maeve, 1992). No information was provided about how this compared to predesign documentation.

Although the report of this redesign evaluation is limited in terms of information about research methods and the measures used to assure rigor of and rationale for data collection, the report highlights one of the important distinctions required with organizational redesign research: the need for defining process and outcome indicators.

Data collected during the medical record review for this study gave indication of change in care delivery *process*, which may or may not have been an anticipated *outcome* of the redesign. In some redesign initiatives, the anticipated outcome may be change in the process of care delivery, which appears to be the case in this study. This initial outcome is then expected to result in some long-term outcome in the recipients of the care delivery practice. Model developers and evaluators using this approach should clearly identify when and how the variables will be differentiated as to their process and outcome aspects.

Counte, Glandon, Oleske, and Hill (1992) conducted a second-order redesign evaluation of the effect of a total quality management (TQM) program on employee job satisfaction and perception of organizational climate and work environment. This study, which was conducted 2 years after the redesign process was initiated, was one of the few in which a sufficiently long period passed between institution of redesign initiative and the collection of outcome data.

In this study of a large Midwest academic medical center, 7,382 employees were surveyed 2 years post–TQM implementation about their perceptions of the work environment. Approximately 71% of employees responded to the questionnaire, of whom 48.6% reported some involvement in the TQM program (29.5% reported no involvement, and 16.0% were uncertain of involvement).

The questionnaire used in the survey contained scales derived from previously tested instruments as well as some developed specifically for the study. Internal consistency reliability estimates for the scales ranged from .49 for job risk and responsibility to .78 for organizational climate and .82 for job satisfaction (Counte et al., 1992).

When responses to subscales were controlled for by differences in individual attributes of respondents, significant differences were seen between those who had participated in the TQM program and those who had not. Those who had participated reported significantly higher levels of general, intrinsic, and extrinsic job satisfaction. Those who had participated also reported more favorable perceptions about support, standards, and identity aspects of organizational climate. Perceptions about the organization were consistently more favorable for those who participated in the TQM process. They perceived the institution to be a desirable place to work and were more likely to recommend the institution to others and to remain employed there. As expected, those who had participated in the TQM process were more often in agreement with the principles of TQM that focused on emphasis on the patient, involvement in decision making, and teamwork (Counte et al., 1992).

A second-order redesign evaluation of a nurse accountability program was reported by Ethridge (1987). In this redesign project, a systematic program was introduced to improve nurses' professional accountability within the institution. The program was introduced in a hospital in which a self-governance model was already in place. New aspects of the accountability program included introduction of a credentialing program, a move to salaried status for all professional nurses, implementation of a spiritual, holistic framework for care delivery, development of a patient acuity billing system, movement of care delivery practices into the home, and introduction of case managers prepared at the baccalaureate level and supported by associate-degree RNs.

Evaluation of the program's success was measured through assessment of RN job stress and job satisfaction. Data were collected prior to the model's implementation and twice following. The actual time frame for postimplementation data collection was unclear because years were used to denote when data were collected but there was no reference for how these related to the actual timing of model implementation or whether the model was partially or fully implemented at the time. Instruments used to collect data were chosen from previous studies of nurse satisfaction and job stress.

In the report of findings, data collected from 11 units surveyed before the redesign process were compared to other units in the hospital and to findings for the same units after the redesign process was undertaken. Significant differences were noted for feelings of competence for units participating in the redesign between baseline and first measurement postimplementation. According to information provided, data for the study units were comparable to data for all units at the first measurement period postimplementation. Satisfaction with time to do the job, quality of care, interaction cohesion, and job enjoyment were significantly greater for study units and for all units after program implementation. This finding may have been an indication of the redesign's effect being observed throughout the institution. On the other hand, because no information was provided about the comparability of the other units to the original 11, the findings also may have been the result of something other than the redesign initiative. This perspective is reinforced by the absence of significant findings at the second data-collection point.

The report of this redesign model highlights two concerns with the reporting of redesign initiatives. First, the redesign initiative was composed of several interdependent components, yet no information was provided about how each of these was assessed individually or collectively for effect. This problem was evident in the labeling of the units involved as pilot sites as "precredentialing units," which appears to focus on only one aspect of the redesign program. Whether or not the other components of the redesign were instituted is unknown, and the labeling of the units as precredentialing suggests that this was the focus of the redesign initiative. The second issue pertains to comparing individual nurses' scores at different times, when different nurses may have comprised the study unit sample. Although using the unit as the unit of analysis has been proposed by Verran, Mark, and Lamb (1992), the researcher should provide some indication of what percentage of the original nurse subjects were included in the samples for the second and third data-collection points. Moreover, some indication of attention to individual versus unit level of analysis should be included in the discussion.

The effect of a day-treatment redesign initiative on patient outcomes was reported by Dickey et al. (1989) and Gudeman et al. (1985). In this redesign process, patients requiring inpatient psychiatric services were admitted to one of two day hospitals in which care delivery was overseen by treatment teams composed of psychiatric health care professionals. Patients who were able to do so left the centers on evenings and weekends; those who were not were housed in an "inn" located within the health care facility. The inn served primarily as a transitional residence rather than a treatment center, although necessary medications and some programs were offered. For patients too ill to stay at the inn, inpatient intensive care unit services were provided. These patients were overseen by the day-treatment team, which worked to stabilize the acute event and return the patient to the day hospital (Gudeman et al., 1985).

The effect of the program was measured by comparing medical records of patients treated 19 months before the program and 19 months after the program was implemented. Characteristics of patients admitted during these two periods were comparable. As expected, the number of patients treated during the day increased following initiation of the program, whereas the number of patients requiring residential care declined from 81% to 56%. Median length of stay was reduced following introduction of the day-treatment program, although not significantly. Readmission rates did not change. Patient safety was not adversely affected by the redesign; patient-related staff accidents, escapes, and use of seclusion and restraints declined significantly (Gudeman et al., 1985).

Per admission costs and total annual costs for patients also were assessed. Introduction of the day-treatment model resulted in per episode inpatient cost reductions of 31% when day hospital inn costs were included in the cost estimation. An assessment for evidence of cost shifting found no indication that reduction in costs associated with use of day care facilities resulted in movement of costs to other agencies or services (Dickey et al., 1989).

Warner (1993) and Warner and Welch (1993) described a redesign evaluation of a milieu enhancement model implemented in a residential home serving approximately 44 orphaned, abandoned, or disadvantaged children. Milieu enhancement strategies included child care worker support groups, increased in-service offerings, completion of admission physicals, and changes in organizational policy.

A cost-effective analysis was conducted as part of this evaluation to determine the effect of the model on children's health status, academic performance, and sex-related behaviors. Data collected at the end of each of the 4 years of the project were compared to preintervention data and to data obtained from a control site comparable in size, affiliation, and services.

Findings showed no differences in mean number of failed grades between experimental and control sites. Differences also were not seen within the experimental site for any years of the project, although differences were seen within the control site. Significantly more subjects failed in Year 3 compared to Year 2. Significant within-group changes were seen for the experimental site for reading, language, and mathematics scores obtained on standard school-administered tests. Comparable information for the control group was not provided (Warner, 1993).

No differences were seen for sex-related beliefs and values between experimental and comparison groups. Beliefs and values change scores increased significantly for the experimental group over time, whereas control group scores declined. Significant differences also were seen for sex-related activities and for frequency of discussions concerning sex-related behaviors. Improvements over time were seen for the experimental group but not for the control group.

Health status was measured by frequency of absences from school and number of dental caries. This last measurement was in response to the inclusion of a fluoride program in the milieu enhancement model. Children from the experimental site missed significantly fewer school days than did children from the control site. No differences were seen for number of caries (Warner, 1993).

The cost of health care provided to children in the milieu enhancement model was computed by adding direct and indirect costs. Indirect cost components were determined through use of daily records kept by child care workers. Because of concerns over completeness and accuracy of recordings, the investigators elected to randomly select 1 month during the summer and 1 month during the academic year to request recordings. These were then multiplied by 3 for the summer month and by nine for the academic month to compute an annual cost figure (Warner & Welch, 1993). Despite the costs associated with services provided by the project, for every $1 of expenditure, the project generated $10.50 worth of benefits, whereas the control site generated $.95 worth of benefits during a comparable period.

One final study that appears to fall into the second-order redesign category is that of Olson and Tetrick (1988), in which they measured the effect of mandated "externally imposed organizational restructuring" (p. 377) on perceived quantitative role overload, interaction/relationship with supervisor, perceived role clarity, overall job satisfaction, and satisfaction with supervision and security. Specifics of the redesign initiative were not included in the report. Consequently, the implications of the study are ambiguous.

In this study, a random sample of subjects was surveyed immediately prior to and 3 months after restructuring concerning attitudes about the job. Scales used in the study were selected from existing satisfaction surveys used within the institution, and reliability estimates were acceptable. Because the preintervention survey was distributed after information about the upcoming redesign had been shared, the researchers have labeled this data point as the "anticipation period" of redesign (Olson & Tetrick, 1988). They did not comment on the fact that because information was shared and employees were in a state of anticipation that a true baseline assessment of perceptions was not achieved.

After controlling for organizational tenure and organizational level, organizational restructuring was not found to be associated with role clarity, role overload, relationship with supervisor, or job satisfaction. Organizational restructuring was associated with job security, although the researchers questioned the practical significance of this finding. The moderating effect of organizational tenure and level were uncertain, with findings showing variability only for those respondents with less than 1 year's tenure in the job. An important issue with this study was the reporting of significant findings for individuals with less than 1 year's tenure at the time of postredesign data collection. Because this data point was 14 months after baseline data were collected, none of these individuals would have been present when baseline data were gathered. Consequently, their responses may have been a reflection of the newness of the job rather than any reaction to organizational redesign.

Studies of Third-Order Redesign

A comprehensive process and initial outcome evaluation of one third-order redesign project was published in 1994 in the *Milbank Quarterly*. In this report, a nine-city community redesign project targeted for persons with chronic mental illness was reviewed (Goldman, Morrissey, & Ridgely, 1990; Morrissey et al., 1994). The purpose of this multicity redesign was to reduce fragmentation and discontinuity in care delivery to clients. The redesign approach involved a two-level process in which case management was used as a mechanism for improving individual-level care; administrative and community co-operative arrangements were used at the systems level to improve services to clients in need.

Qualitative and quantitative methods were used to assess the extent of the redesign on client outcomes. Key informants were used to determine whether the redesign was meeting the needs of the chronically mentally ill. To assess for early versus late performance of the redesign, a questionnaire was distributed at the beginning and the end of the project (Morrissey et al., 1994). Unfortunately, no information was provided about how this tool was developed or tested for reliability and validity. Interviews of staff were conducted to determine the extent to which interagency relationships were becoming more coordinated and centralized. In addition, quantitative measures were used to capture comparable data for density, centralization, and fragmentation of services. Again, no information was included about psychometric testing for these indexes. Perceptions of key informants suggested that ability to influence change was most effective at the local mental health agency level and less so at the community support services level.

This study also exemplified the process as outcome measurement concern. Researchers used an outcome measure of program effectiveness (density, centralization, and fragmentation of services) as a process component of the redesign model, one that was expected to improve client outcome. The study also highlighted the difficulties associated with measuring the "true" effect of an intervention. At the same time the study redesign model was focusing on fiscal incentives to decentralize services, so were the states in which the study was conducted (Frank & Gaynor, 1994). Consequently, whether the changes seen in outcomes were the result of the redesign or the state's financial incentives is unknown.

Continuity of care and client outcomes were measured through longitudinal data collection from two cohorts of clients (Lehman, Postrado, Roth, McNary, & Goldman, 1994; Shern et al., 1994), families, and care providers (Shern et al., 1994). Cohorts were selected from two periods in the redesign process: 2 years after initial funding and 4 years after funding. Continuity of care, which was defined as "same case manager," differed according to group at 2 months postdischarge. The second cohort, which was expected to be more strongly affected by the redesign process, had significantly higher scores for continuity of care. These differences disappeared by 1 year, however (Lehman et al., 1994). At 12 months, a significant effect was seen by site. Site of the redesign initiative also appeared to influence frequency of change in case manager.

The reasons for the differences by site are unclear. One plausible explanation could be differences in extent of redesign, as characteristics of the subjects in cohorts were described as comparable. If the extent of the redesign initiative varied across sites, differences in outcome would be likely. Unfortunately, no measure of extent of redesign intervention was included. Consequently, the effect of this factor on redesign outcome is uncertain.

No noticeable effect was seen as a result of case manager oversight or involvement in the project as a whole (Lehman et al., 1994). Quality of life and satisfaction with care delivery were unchanged over time, whereas reports of unmet client needs varied according to site. In one site the redesign project appeared to seriously disrupt the ongoing functioning of the system, resulting in dissatisfaction and negative perception about benefit (Shern et al., 1994).

A second study of a third-order redesign initiative compared the costs of three types of residential options for the care of severely mentally disabled adults (Galster, Champney, & Williams, 1994). In this study, costs associated with serving clients in three types of residential settings (public or subsidized private rental dwellings, unsubsidized private rental dwellings, and state psychiatric hospital) were compared. The study was initiated following the introduction of a demonstration project designed to provide housing supports for severely mentally disabled adults, which included the availability of mobile crisis and case management teams.

Data for this evaluation were collected through monthly interviews of approximately 48% of eligible clients. Data pertaining to mental, physical, and dental services obtained, out-of-pocket expenses incurred, housing expenses, personal income, employment, and volunteer work were collected.

Costs of institutionalized care delivered at the state hospital were significantly greater than costs at any of the other residential treatment options. An unexpected finding in this study was an increase in overall costs for subsidized housing. When subsidies were provided, clients tended to rent more expensive apartments. Because clients in this study were not randomly assigned to type of residence, findings may have been influenced by individual characteristics in addition to type of residence (Galster et al., 1994). Nonetheless, with costs in excess of $4,200 to $5,300 per client per month for state hospital placements, the findings provide support for the deinstitutionalization of mentally ill adults.

A third study categorized here as third-order was reported by Olden and Johnson (1993). It is included because it involved the redesign of one hospital's care delivery approach for mentally ill patients, although the program itself was directed by the Kaiser Foundation Health Plan. In this redesign process the Kaiser Foundation contracted for inpatient psychiatric services with a general hospital containing a 22-bed locked psychiatric ward.

The redesign approach involved contracting with seven private-practice psychiatrists who provided services to the health plan's clients. A reimbursement formula for care of these patients was calculated and included laboratory studies, services, and medications. In addition, a regional manager for the health plan was located on site and participated in discussions about individual patient care needs. This process of working directly with the regional manager was defined as a "facilitated" approach, in which rapid identification of problems likely to prolong length of stay was expected.

Over the 5-year period during which the redesign was initiated, costs per admission were reduced by 47%. Readmission rate within 60 days of discharge was 16.9%, which was higher than expected. Patient satisfaction measured by survey was reported as favorable, with 91% of respondents reporting being very or extremely satisfied with care (Olden & Johnson, 1993). Unfortunately, no information was provided about the reliability and validity of the satisfaction instrument used, nor was there any information about how the data from this sample compared with other samples of comparable patients.

DISCUSSION

Comprehensive studies of organizational redesign and its effect on outcomes are few. The majority of the studies reported were focused on segments within the organization rather than the organization as a whole. In addition, findings tend to be inconsistent, although some patterns do emerge.

Job satisfaction findings are mixed, with some studies noting intermittent and partial change (Zelauskas & Howes, 1992) and others finding little or none (Ethridge, 1987; Garfink et al., 1991). What has been found to occur, however, is improved perception of the work group (Garfink et al., 1991; Weisman et al., 1993). These findings suggested that the early effect of organizational redesign may be a change in perception of the desirability and value of the work group and work environment, which subsequently leads to increased overall work satisfaction.

Studies of the effect of redesign initiatives on cost to the institution suggested that models directed toward increased collaboration and professional staff accountability are no more costly than are other care delivery models (Wong et al., 1993). These models also resulted in cost savings related to reduced turnover and decreased need for supplemental staff (Malloch, Milton, & Jobes, 1990). Redesign models in which professional staff were replaced by nonprofessional staff also appear to result in short-term cost savings (Garfink et al., 1991). Whether these early savings are offset by long-term increases in costs associated with quality of care outcomes is unknown.

The review of articles concerning organizational redesign and outcomes has uncovered a problem needing close attention in the future. Reports of organizational redesign tend to include anecdotal information concerning extent of effect. This may be due to failure to conduct comprehensive outcome evaluations or to the publication standards of the journals in which organizational redesign articles are published. One of the essential components of a comprehensive program evaluation is the presentation of findings useful for policymakers and decision makers. Many of the articles reviewed for this analysis were contained in journals targeted for practitioners and administrators (e.g., *The Journal of Nursing Administration*), where a focus on applicability of findings is expected. Because of the application focus of these journals, less attention may be paid to study designs and issues of scientific rigor. This is a problem, especially for individuals seeking data-based reports on which to build theory and further study. In future, articles addressing both focuses are needed: those targeted for practitioners and policymakers, where application of findings are stressed, and those targeted for researchers, where methods and analyses are the focus.

An additional problem identified during the review is the limited information provided about the condition of the organizational environment prior to redesign. Absent are descriptions of any comprehensive assessment of the environment and efforts made to assess how data collected retrospectively may have been influenced by an entirely different set of organizational characteristics. For example, in a report of a care partnerships model (Schroeder & Maeve, 1992), no information was provided about how the chart review data compared to prior documentation standards or what those preimplementation standards were.

Future studies of organizational redesign also should incorporate some measure for controlling for the effects of individual, environmental, and organizational characteristics because differences in patient outcome may be the result of preexisting characteristics (Daley et al., 1988) or method of assessing illness severity (Iezzoni, 1989) rather than intervention or activity during hospitalization. Outcomes also may be influenced by subtle, undefined differences in processes of care delivery relating to method of payment (Bull, 1988). Without specific information about these factors, no conclusion can be made about reports of positive or negative redesign outcome.

Follow-up work needs to be done to determine whether hospitals with high nurse-to-patient ratios and all-RN or predominantly RN staff continue to report highly satisfied, committed employees. In many of the redesign models proposed by hospitals today, programs and characteristics associated with hospitals of excellence in the past (Fuszard, Green, Kujala, & Talley, 1994; Kramer & Schmalenberg, 1988; Mitchell, Armstrong, Simpson, & Lentz, 1989) are being altered or eliminated. Early reports (Ingersoll, 1995) suggest that redesign models incorporating increased numbers of nonprofessional staff are being received with mixed reaction as to their desirability and effectiveness. Moreover, there are no longitudinal studies demonstrating the effect of these mixed staffing models on patient care or cost to institution. Although early cost savings through use of less expensive staff are being reported, no information is available about how patient-related events and time spent in delegation activities affect cost estimations.

Identification of reliable and valid outcome measures also should be included as a research priority for the future. At this time there is little information available about which are the most useful indicators of change, particularly where nursing interventions are concerned. Multiple measures will be required; blended measures in which combined quality-of-care scores are used or outcome indexes are computed from multiple indicators will be problematic. Future studies also will require a multidimensional approach, making these studies complex and costly.

Researchers of organizational redesign will need to pay close attention to extent of redesign intervention. Failure to assess extent of redesign may result in what has been referred to as Type III evaluation error. In Type III error, the intervention is not introduced as intended or is not measured as introduced (Basch, Sliepcevich, Gold, Duncan, & Kolbe, 1985; Carlson, 1977). It occurs when the intervention introduced differs from the intervention planned, when the "amount" of intervention is not sufficient to produce an effect, and when the intervention does not address the underlying problem for which it was intended. To reduce the potential for this problem, some measure of extent of model implementation is needed.

Inclusion of a process component to the overall evaluation plan also is required, as this aspect of the evaluation provides information about what is done, how it is done, and whether or not what was intended is accomplished. Some researchers have begun to introduce process evaluation methods into their studies (Ingersoll, Bazar, & Zentner, 1993; Taft, Jones, & Minch, 1992), but the formal inclusion of process evaluation steps and methods for quantifying the extent of organizational redesign continue to be the exception rather than the rule. This situation is particularly troublesome for studies such as the one reported by Barhyte et al. (1987), in which the number of units involved is small and then only a portion of the units succeed in fully accomplishing the redesign in initiative.

CONCLUSION

Considerable research is needed to clarify the effect of first-, second-, and third-order organizational redesign on institutional and consumer outcomes. Well-designed studies are needed in which different organizational models are tested. Both qualitative and quantitative approaches are appropriate, with attention paid to both process and outcome components of the redesign evaluation. Unless empirical evidence is available to support decisions made about organizational structure, health care agencies are likely to suffer the same limited experiences reported in analyses of large corporations where initiatives were instituted earlier (Hall, Rosenthal, & Wade, 1993).

REFERENCES

Barhyte, D. Y., Counte, M. D., & Christman, L. P. (1987). Effects of decentralization on job attendance. *Nursing Administration Quarterly, 11*(4), 37–46.

Basch, C. E., Sliepcevich, E. M., Gold, R. S., Duncan, D. F., & Kolbe, L. J. (1985). Avoiding Type III errors in health education program evaluations: A case study. *Health Education Quarterly, 12*, 315–331.

Bray, M. L., & Edwards, L. H. (1994). A primary health care approach using Hispanic outreach workers as nurse extenders. *Public Health Nursing, 11*, 7–11.

Brett, J. L. L., & Tonges, M. C. (1990). Restructured patient care delivery: Evaluation of the ProACT model. *Nursing Economics, 8*, 36–44.

Brooten, D., Kumar, S., Brown, L. P., Butts, P., Finkler, S. A., Bakewell-Sachs, S., Gibbons, A., & Delivoria-Papadopoulos, M. (1986). A randomized clinical trial of early hospital discharge and home follow-up of very low birth weight infants. *New England Journal of Medicine, 315*, 934–939.

Bull, M. J. (1988). Influence of diagnosis-related groups on discharge planning, professional practice, and patient care. *Journal of Professional Nursing, 4*, 415–421.

Carlson, W. A. (1977). The measurement of outcome evaluation. In G. R. Gilbert & P. J. Conklin (Eds.), *Evaluation management: A sourcebook of readings* (pp. 146–184). Charlottesville, VA: Federal Executive Institute.

Cassard, S. D., Weisman, C. S., Gordon, D. L., & Wong, R. (1994). The impact of unit-based self-management by nurses on patient outcomes. *Health Services Research, 29*, 415–433.

Cassidy, J. (1992). Patient-focused delivery promises to reshape hospitals. *Hospital Progress, 73*(4), 20–24.

Clark, M. F., & Zornow, R. A. (1989). Nursing organizing systems: A comparative study. *Western Journal of Nursing Research, 11*, 757–764.

Counte, M. A., Glandon, G. L., Oleske, D. M., & Hill, J. P. (1992). Total quality management in a health care organization: How are employees affected? *Hospital and Health Services Administration, 37*, 503–518.

Daley, J., Jencks, S., Draper, D., Lenhart, G., Thomas, N., Walker, J. (1988). Predicting hospital-associated mortality for Medicare patients. *Journal of the American Medical Association, 260*, 3617–3624.

Dear, M. R., Weisman, C. S., & O'Keefe, S. (1985). Evaluation of a contract model for professional nursing practice. *Health Care Management Review, 10*(2), 65–77.

Dickey, B., Binner, P. R., Leff, S., Uyeda, M. K., Schlesinger, M. J., & Gudeman, J. E. (1989). Containing mental health treatment costs through program design: A Massachusetts study. *American Journal of Public Health, 79*, 863–867.

Dienemann, J., & Gessner, T. (1992). Restructuring nursing care delivery systems. *Nursing Economics, 10*, 253–258.

Ethridge, P. (1987). Nurse accountability program improves satisfaction, turnover. *Health Progress, 68*(4), 44–49.

Fleishman, J. A., Mor, V., & Piette, J. (1991). AIDS case management: The client's perspective. *Health Services Research, 26*, 447–470.

Frank, R. G., & Gaynor, M. (1994). Fiscal decentralization of public mental health care and the Robert Wood Johnson Foundation program on chronic mental illness. *Milbank Quarterly, 72*, 81–104.

Fuszard, B., Green, E., Kujala, E., & Talley, B. (1994). Rural magnet hospitals of excellence: Part 1. *Journal of Nursing Administration, 24*(1), 21–26.

Galster, G. C., Champney, T. F., & Williams, Y. (1994). Costs of caring for persons with long-term mental illness in alternative residential settings. *Evaluation and Program Planning, 17*, 239–248.

Garfink, C. M., Kirby, K. K., Bachman, S. S., & Starck, P. (1991). The University Hospital Nurse Extender Model: Part 3. Program evaluation. *Journal of Nursing Administration, 21*(3), 21–27.

Goldman, H. H., Morrissey, J. P., & Ridgely, M. S. (1990). Form and function of mental health authorities at RWJ Foundation program sites: Preliminary observations. *Hospital and Community Psychiatry, 417* 1222–1230.

Gudeman, J. E., Dickey, B., Evans, A., & Shore, M. F. (1985). Four-year assessment of a day hospital-inn program as an alternative to inpatient hospitalization. *American Journal of Psychiatry, 142*, 1330–1333. A)

Hall, G., Rosenthal, J., & Wade, J. (1993). How to make reengineering really work. *Harvard Business Review, 71*(6), 119–131.

Hunter, D. E. K., Buick, W. P., Wellington, T., & Dzerovych, G. (1993). Initial evaluation of reorganized hospitalization services in a community mental health center. *Hospital and Community Psychiatry, 44*, 271–275.

Ingersoll, G. L., (1995). Licensed practical nurses in critical care areas: Intensive care unit nurses' perceptions about the role. *Heart and Lung, 24*, 83–88.

Ingersoll, G. L., Bazar, M., & Zentner, J. (1993). Monitoring unit-based innovations: A process evaluation approach, *Nursing Economics, 11*, 137–143.

Iezzoni, L. I. (1989). Using severity information for quality assessment: A review of three cases by five severity measures. *Quality Review Bulletin, 15*, 376–382.

James, I., Milne, D. L., & Firth, H. (1990). A systematic comparison of feedback and staff discussion in changing the ward atmosphere. *Journal of Advanced Nursing, 15*, 329–336.

Jones, W. J., & Bullard, M. (1993). Translating operational change into facility design. *Healthcare Forum Journal, 36*(1), 67–69.

Kramer, M., & Schmalenberg, C. (1988). Magnet hospitals: Part 1. Institutions of excellence. *Journal of Nursing Administration, 18*(1), 18–24.

Lehman, A. F., Postrado, L. T., Roth, D., McNary, S. W., & Goldman, H. H. (1994). Continuity of care and client outcomes in the Robert Wood Johnson Foundation program on chronic mental illness. *Milbank Quarterly, 72*, 105–122.

Malloch, K. M., Milton, D. A., & Jobes, M. O. (1990). A model for differentiated nursing practice. *Journal of Nursing Administration, 20*(2), 20–25

Mamon, J., Steinwachs, D. M., Fahey, M., Bone, L. R., Oktay, J., & Klein, L. (1992). Impact of hospital discharge planning on meeting patient needs after returning home. *Health Services Research, 27*, 155–175.

McCorkle, R., Jepson, C., Malone, D., Lusk, E., Braitman, L., Buhler-Wilkerson, K.,

& Daly, J. (1994). The impact of posthospital home care on patients with cancer. *Research in Nursing and Health, 17*, 243–251.

Meyer, A. D., Goes, J. B., & Brooks, G. R. (1993). Organizations reacting to hyperturbulence. In G. P. Huber & W. H. Glick (Eds.), *Organizational change and redesign: Ideas and insights for improving performance* (pp. 66–111). New York: Oxford University Press.

Mitchell, P. H., Armstrong, S., Simpson, T. F., & Lentz, M. (1989). American Association of Critical-Care Nurses Demonstration Project: Profile of excellence in critical care nursing. *Heart and Lung, 18*, 219–237.

Morrissey, J. P., Calloway, M., Bartko, W. T., Ridgely, M. S., Goldman, H. H., & Paulson, R. I. (1994). Local mental health authorities and service system change: Evidence from the Robert Wood Johnson Foundation program on chronic mental illness. *Milbank Quarterly, 72*, 49–80.

Olden, K. W., & Johnson, M. P. (1993). A "facilitated" model of inpatient psychiatric care. *Hospital and Community Health, 44*, 879–882.

Olson, D. A., & Tetrick, L. E. (1988). Organizational restructuring: The impact on role perceptions, work relationship, and satisfaction. *Group and Organization Studies, 13*, 374–388.

Schroeder, C., & Maeve, M. K. (1992). Nursing care partnerships at the Denver Nursing Project in Human Caring: An application and extension of caring theory in practice. *Advances in Nursing Science, 15*(2), 25–38.

Shern, D. L., Wilson, N. Z., Coen, A. S., Patrick, D. C., Foster, M., Bartsch, D. A., & Demmler, J. (1994). Client outcomes: 2. Longitudinal client data from the Colorado treatment outcome study. *Milbank Quarterly, 72*, 123–148.

Shortell, S. M., Morrison, E. M., & Friedman, B. (1992). *Strategic choices for America's hospitals: Managing change in turbulent times.* San Francisco: Jossey-Bass.

Taft, S. H., Jones, P. K., & Minch, E. L. (1992). Strengthening hospital nursing: Part 3. Differences among professional groups in the hospital planning process. *Journal of Nursing Administration, 22*(7/8), 41–50.

Teresi, J., Holmes, D., Benenson, E., Monaco, C., Barrett, V., & Koren, M. J. (1992). Evaluation of primary care nursing in long-term care. *Research on Aging, 15*, 414–432.

Verran, J. A., Mark, B. A., & Lamb, G. (1992). Psychometric examination of instruments using aggregated data. *Research in Nursing and Health 15*, 237–240.

Vines, S. W., & Williams-Burgess, C. (1994). Effects of a community health nursing parent-baby (ad)venture program on depression and other selected maternal-child health outcomes. *Public Health Nursing, 11*, 188–195.

Warner, S. (1993). The cost-effectiveness of a nursing demonstration project: Part 2. *Archives of Psychiatric Nursing, 7*, 61–67.

Warner, S., & Welch, R. (1993). The cost-benefits of a nursing demonstration project: Part 3. *Archives of Psychiatric Nursing, 7*, 68–73.

Weisman, C. S., Gordon, D. L., Cassard, S. D., Bergner, M., & Wong, R. (1993). The effects of unit self-management on hospital nurses' work process, work satisfaction, and retention. *Medical Care, 31*, 381–393.

Wong, R., Gordon, D. L., Cassard, S. D., Weisman, C. S., & Bergner, M. (1993). A cost analysis of a professional practice model for nursing. *Nursing Economics, 11*, 292–297.

Zelauskas, B., & Howes, D. G. (1992). The effects of implementing a professional practice model. *Journal of Nursing Administration, 22*(7/8), 18–23.

Chapter 7

Organizational Culture

BARBARA A. MARK
SCHOOL OF NURSING
MEDICAL COLLEGE OF VIRGINIA
VIRGINIA COMMONWEALTH UNIVERSITY

CONTENTS

This chapter includes a review of the research on organizational culture in the nursing and other health services literature published since 1985. Notwithstanding the frequency with which the concept of culture occurs in the popular management literature, there is, in fact, a dearth of empirical studies in both the nursing and the health services literature. Substantive theoretical development of the concept of organizational culture has occurred in the organizational literature rather than in the nursing or health services literature; the richness of this theoretical development, however, is not reflected in the published research in nursing or elsewhere in health care. Therefore, the chapter begins with a review of this theoretical literature, particularly as it relates to the definition of organizational culture. Next, the empirical studies in nursing and in health services research are described. Then conceptual and methodological issues that must be addressed in organizational culture research are discussed. Finally, recommendations for future research on organizational culture in nursing and health services are presented.

SOURCES OF DATA

This chapter reviews articles published from 1985 to 1994. A computer search of MEDLINE and CD-ROM Cumulative Index to Nursing and Allied Health Literature (CINAHL) was conducted using the following keywords: organizational culture, culture, corporate culture. In addition, a manual search of the *Journal of Nursing Administration, Nursing Administration Quarterly, Image: The Journal of Nursing Scholarship, Nursing Economics, Nursing Research, Western Journal of Nursing Research*, and *Research in Nursing and Health* was also conducted for the same period. Studies were included if they (a) were published in English, (b) focused on organizational culture (not organizational climate),[1] (c) used hospitals rather than educational institutions as the focal unit, and (d) reported empirical data, regardless of whether it was qualitative or quantitative. Although numerous articles were found in which authors explored the implications of the concept of organizational culture for nursing and health care, they were excluded from this review because they were not empirically based. Unpublished doctoral dissertations also were excluded.

ORGANIZATIONAL CULTURE: THE CONCEPT

Reichers and Schneider (1990) suggested that concept development proceeds through an evolutionary process that encompasses three stages. The first stage, introduction and elaboration, occurs when a concept is "invented, discovered, or borrowed from another field" (p. 6). This stage can be identified by attempts to explain to a largely "naive" audience the definition of the concept, its importance, and particularly its worth in promoting the understanding of previously disparate findings. During the second stage, labeled evaluation and augmentation, critical reviews begin to appear that address problems in conceptualization, method, and conflicting or equivocal results. As a result of these reviews, extensions and enhancements of prior work tend to appear. In the final stage, consolidation and accommodation, definitional diversity decreases, with researchers generally tending toward one or two generally well-accepted definitions. Antecedents and consequences are well known, and operationalization is no longer controversial. As will become apparent from this review, the development of the concept of organizational culture still resides in the first stage. In fact, one writer (Mumby, 1994) suggests that organizational culture research in the past 10 years has been both a blessing and a curse.

It is generally acknowledged that the term "organizational culture" first appeared in the literature in a 1979 *Administrative Science Quarterly* article by Pettigrew. In that article, Pettigrew attempted to use the concepts developed in sociology and anthropology to understand "how purpose, commitment, and order are created in the early life of an organization" (p. 572), in this case, a British boarding school. He defined culture as "the system of such publicly and collectively accepted meanings operating for a given group at a given time. This system of terms, forms, categories, and images interprets a people's own situation to themselves" (p. 574). Pettigrew, however, critiqued his own definition, suggesting that culture should be understood as a "family" of concepts: symbol, language, ideology, belief, ritual and myth, with symbol being the most inclusive category.

There are essentially two approaches to the study of organizational culture: as something the organization *has* or as something the organization *is* (Smircich, 1983). Another way of describing this distinction is that in the former case, which is primarily a functionalist orientation, an organization is understood as a social system exhibiting a variety of cultural attributes; whereas in the latter case, which is primarily an interpretivist orientation, an organization is perceived holistically as the cultural manifestation of a social system. In the functionalist orientation, the interest tends to focus on understanding the relationships among culture, leadership, structure, and strategy with the goal of improving organizational effectiveness or assisting a manager in the process of organizational change. In the interpretivist orientation, the interest is in studying social significance, "how things, events, and interactions come to be meaningful" (Smircich, 1985, p. 63). The goal of the organizational interpretivist is "interpreting, decoding and deconstructing the meaning of organization in the modern age" (Smircich, 1985, p. 67).

From the functionalist perspective, culture is something the organization has—a variable, independent or dependent, depending on the researcher's interest. Culture can be considered as something imported into the organization through personnel, environment, or technology or as a variable internal to the organization. In the latter case, culture is usually defined as the "glue" that holds the organization together or as the values of organization members, expressed in a variety of symbolic devices such as myths, stories, rituals, heroes, and legends. When the organization's rules are examined from the functionalist perspective, it is the *content* of the rules that is of interest, rather than the process by which social meaning is given expression in those rules. Although there is no singular definition of culture arising from the perspective of culture as variable, there does seem to be a consistent theme woven through these definitions: Culture is a "common set of shared meanings or understandings about the group/organization and its problems, goals, and practices" (Reichers & Schneider, 1990, p. 23).

When organizational culture is conceptualized as something the organization is—that is, as "root metaphor"—it suggests a view of organizations as "expressive forms" and as "manifestations of human consciousness" (Smircich, 1983, p. 347). In research stemming from this perspective, investigators explore the "phenomenon of organization as subjective experience" (Smircich, 1983, p. 348). Within the conceptualization of culture as root metaphor, three distinct perspectives can be identified: the cognitive, the symbolic and the psychodynamic.

The cognitive perspective derives from ethnoscience, a branch of cognitive anthropology. Within the cognitive perspective, culture is a "system of shared cognitions or a system of knowledge and beliefs" (Smircich, 1983, p. 348). When researchers from this perspective investigate the organization's rules, the focus tends to be on the *process* by which rules, as organized patterns of thought, come to be the expression of a group's "unconscious logic" (Smircich, 1983, p. 348), which then serves to guide action. In the symbolic perspective, culture is a "pattern of symbolic discourse," understood through an examination of the ways in which experience becomes meaningful to people in organizations and of how this meaning guides their behavior. In the psychodynamic perspective, organizations are seen as the expression of unconscious psychodynamic processes. Research on organizational culture from the psychodynamic perspective is focused on uncovering hidden but universal dimensions of the human mind (Smircich, 1983). Clearly, no single conceptualization of culture emerges when culture is considered as root metaphor.

As will be evidenced in the discussion to follow, although nursing research and health services research have tended to approach research on organizational culture by focusing on rules, there has been little theoretical discussion of the conceptual basis of this approach. In addition, the implications of nursing and health services research indicate that researchers treat culture as variable, that which may be controlled by managers in efforts to introduce organizational change or to improve organizational functioning.

NURSING AND HEALTH SERVICES RESEARCH ON ORGANIZATIONAL CULTURE

The first article in the nursing literature that focused on organizational culture appeared in 1986. In this nonempirical article,[2] del Bueno and Vincent (1986) used the Wilkins (1983) definition of culture: "the combination of the symbols, language, assumptions and behaviors that overtly manifest an organization's norms and values . . . the taken-for-granted and shared meanings people assign to their social surrounds that can have a profound effect on an organization's decision making and performance" (p. 15). This definition is consistent with the view of culture as variable, in this case as internal variable. The balance of the article focused on levels of culture, the use of organizational metaphors (e.g., the military metaphor, the sports/team metaphor) as they have been used to illustrate organizational culture, and organizational transitions in which culture becomes particularly transparent (e.g., when an individual first joins an organization, when there is a change in a chief administrative officer).

Despite the extensiveness of the literature search, few articles reported empirical research on organizational culture in nursing and in health services research literature. Only 12 articles were found that met the inclusion criteria. Their presentation is divided into three sections. The first section describes a series of qualitative articles on organizational culture (Coeling & Simms, 1993a, 1993b; Coeling & Wilcox, 1988, 1990). The second section contains articles that used the Organizational Culture Inventory (OCI; McDaniel & Stumpf, 1993; Shortell, Rousseau, Gillies, Devers, & Simons, 1991; Shortell et al., 1994; Thomas, Ward, Chorba, & Kumiega, 1990; Zimmerman et al., 1993, 1994). The final section contains two additional articles (Fleeger, 1993; Nystrom, 1993) that address other aspects of organizational culture.

Qualitative Research on Organizational Culture

In two articles, Coeling and Wilcox (1988,1990) published the first reports in the nursing literature in which researchers examined empirically the organizational culture of nursing units. In the 1988 report of their ethnographic study, the authors compared the day shift cultures of two medical-surgical units. The authors defined culture as a "set of solutions devised by a group of people to meet specific problems posed by the situations they face in common" (p. 16). Operationally, culture was defined as the work group's rules, "the behaviors . . . that group members consider to be the appropriate responses to given situations" (p. 16). Using participant observation and an ethnographic approach, Coeling and Wilcox (1988) compared two nursing units with regard to their rules for working together, for telling others what to do, for following established standards, for organizing and using time, for taking the patient's perspective and rules for implementing change. The researchers identified important differences between the units in the rules that guided behavior. Coeling and Wilcox (1988) asserted that these differences have management implications with regard to hiring personnel, orienting new staff, facilitating change, and implementing successful teaching strategies.

In the later article (Coeling & Wilcox, 1990) the researchers reported essentially the same data from a somewhat different perspective. In this article the authors suggested that resistance to the implementation of a change in nursing practice model might be explained on the basis of a concomitant but unrecognized change in the organizational culture of the nursing unit. Again, culture was defined as unit rules, but the conceptualization of rules was organized around four anthropological dimensions: individualism/collectivism, physical/psychological aspects, power relationships, and uncertainty/avoidance. Coeling and Wilcox then described elements of primary nursing and examined how well the work rules on the renal/urology unit supported a change from team nursing to a form of primary nursing.

Building on this previous work, Coeling and Simms (1993a, 1993b), in a two-part article, asserted that understanding a nursing unit's culture might assist in the process of introducing a new nursing practice model. The first article described the development of the Nursing Unit Cultural Assessment Tool (NUCAT). This tool contains 50 different cultural behaviors and their associated norms, rated on a 6-point scale. The NUCAT gives a "comprehensive description of nursing unit culture by providing a unit score (mean) for each of the 50 different behaviors" (Coeling & Simms, 1993b, p. 15). Examples of these norms are working in an efficient manner, using individual judgment, being assertive, and being competitive. Coeling and Wilcox's earlier studies (1988, 1990) are cited as part of the process of instrument development. However, those studies dealt with rules, whereas Coeling and Simms (1993a), in the NUCAT, focused on norms. This discrepancy in terminology raises the issue of how rules differ from norms, in both conceptualization and operationalization. For example, rules are generally thought to be explicit, whereas norms are considered to be implicit. Rules are frequently codified as procedures or standards, and they are written, thus allowing public scrutiny. In contrast, norms are communicated through group behavior; deviance from a group norm is often met with social sanctions. A clear conceptual distinction between norms and rules has important implications for the procedures selected to investigate them, as well as for improving construct validity.

In the second part of the article (Coeling & Simms, 1993b), the authors described the use of the NUCAT with 607 members of the nursing staff on 33 nursing units in three health care institutions. Using graphic representations, the authors illustrate some of the key cultural differences among selected units in each of the institutions. They then describe how the information derived from the NUCAT might be used to plan innovations, particularly the introduction of new practice models.

The authors' statement that the items on the NUCAT are independent of each other raises further issues of reliability and validity. For example, the item

"How acceptable is it to be assertive with your coworkers?" seems, at least conceptually, related to the item "How acceptable is it to tell others directly what to do, rather than give them ideas about what they could do?" Without additional information about interitem and item-to-total correlations (and other indicators of reliability), as well as factor analytic results, it is difficult to evaluate fully the psychometric characteristics of the NUCAT.

Research Using the Organizational Culture Inventory

The OCI, developed by Cooke and Lafferty (1989), is frequently used to measure organizational culture and has been extensively evaluated for reliability and validity (Cooke & Rousseau, 1988). The OCI is composed of 12 scales of 10 items each, on a 1-to-5 scale, measuring individuals' perceptions about the ways in which "organizational members are expected to think and behave in relation both to their tasks and to other people" (Cooke & Rousseau, 1988, p. 252). The 12 scales are (a) humanistic-helpful, (b) affiliative, (c) approval, (d) conventional, (e) dependent, (f) avoidance, (g) oppositional, (h) power, (i) competitive, (j) competence/perfectionistic, (k) achievement, and (l) self-actualizing. From these 12 scales, principal components factor analysis yields three underlying dimensions. The first dimension is the people/security culture, characterized by norms for approval, and conventional, dependent, and avoidance styles. The satisfaction culture has norms for achievement, self-actualization, and humanistic-helpful and affiliative styles. The task/security culture has norms for oppositional, power, competitive, and perfectionistic styles (Cooke & Rousseau, 1988). The 12 styles, with their underlying factors, are placed on a circumplex to illustrate visually the culture of the work unit. Cooke and Rousseau (1988) reported alpha reliability coefficients in a sample of 661 individuals (including 526 members of 18 different organizations and 135 participants in executive development or graduate business programs) ranging from .67 for the oppositional scale to .92 for the affiliative scale. Nine of the 12 scales had alphas ≥ .80. Factor analytic results revealed a distinct factor structure, except for the oppositional scale (factor loading of .41 on the people/security factor and .46 on the task/security culture). Overall, the OCI explained 65% of the variance in responses (Cooke & Rousseau, 1988).

Thomas et al. (1990) examined responses to the OCI of 56 nurses in a metropolitan community hospital. The authors first described an "ideal" nursing culture, defined by a "small group of nurses representing several hospitals" (p. 19), as "constructive" [their term for the Cooke and Rousseau (1988) satisfaction culture]. However, in their larger sample, Thomas et al. (1990) found a "weak" culture. In other words, nurses did not report strong norms on any of the 12 styles. In addition, there was little agreement among them about the norms. Compared with the "ideal" culture reported earlier by the authors, these nurses had higher expectations for both the task/security culture (called by these authors the "aggressive/defensive style") and the people security culture (called the "passive/defensive style") and lower expectations for the satisfaction culture (called the "constructive style"). Compared with those in staff nurse positions, nurses in administrative positions reported slightly higher expectations for satisfaction-oriented behaviors such as achievement and self-actualization and substantially stronger expectations for competitive and power behaviors.

This article was the first to appear in the nursing literature using a quantitative approach and a well-validated instrument to measure organizational culture. The authors' purpose, namely, to illustrate how norms can be measured and interpreted, was well served. However, inadequate information was provided about the sample from which the "ideal" nursing culture was derived. Similarly, the authors did not furnish details on selection of the nurses who made up the larger sample, raising the issue of representativeness. And despite the use of an instrument with well-validated psychometric properties, no information on reliability or validity in the authors' sample was provided.

Researchers conducted a longitudinal study of 42 intensive care units (Shortell et al., 1991, 1994; Zimmerman et al., 1993, 1994). They investigated, among other questions, the relationship of organizational culture to a variety of outcomes. In one of the early publications from this research program, Shortell et al. (1991) reported on the construct validity of a 48-item sample from the OCI. In their sample of 2,540 participants (nurses, physicians, unit clerks, top managers), the authors reconfirmed the three factors underlying the OCI scales: the team/satisfaction culture, the people/security culture, and the task/security culture.

Next, Zimmerman et al. (1993) reported results using a subsample of 316 nurses and 202 physicians from nine of the intensive care units (ICUs) included in the larger study. This study examined the relationships among organizational culture, several other independent variables (leadership by nurses and physicians, coordination mechanisms, communication, and collaborative problem solving), risk-adjusted mortality, and length of stay. In general, higher-performing ICUs were characterized by a team satisfaction-oriented culture, whereas lower performing units were concerned with "personal security, procedural issues, hospital rules and bureaucracy" (p. 1446). As the authors of the study were careful to point out, however, these results were not uniform across all nine ICUs. For example, some of the higher-performing units exhibited "poor" cultural practices, and some of the units that performed less well exhibited "excellent" cultural practices. In addition, the authors acknowledge the difficulty that arises from the absence of objective performance criteria.

A more in-depth follow-up, using on-site organizational analysis of two of the nine ICUs described in the previous work by Zimmerman et al. (1994), has also been reported. The two units were selected because one had significantly better than expected mortality and the other experienced significantly worse mortality. However, the relationship between their cultures and outcomes was puzzling. The ICU in which the nursing culture emphasized creativity, undertaking challenging tasks, open communication, and mutual support experienced significantly worse risk-adjusted mortality and mean actual to predicted ICU length of stay. In contrast, the ICU that experienced better mortality and length of stay ratios was characterized by a nursing culture that relied on "positional authority, punishing mistakes, bureaucratic control and avoiding conflict" (p. 134). The physician culture on the worse-performing unit was characterized by the absence of strong behavioral norms, whereas the physician culture on the better-performing unit was "team oriented, emphasizing achievement, self-expression and cooperative relationships, but also stressed approval and conventionality" (p. 134). An interesting observation is that, on both units, there were discrepancies between the cultures of the nurses and the physicians, raising the question about the relative contributions to unit effectiveness of these perhaps conflicting cultures. The results of this study also raise questions for those who suggest that culture management is the primary leverage point for organizational change and improved effectiveness.

A more recent publication reports the results of a theoretically driven examination of the relationship between management processes and a variety of outcomes on the original 42 ICUs. Shortell et al. (1994) found that caregiver interaction, a composite scale composed of measures of unit culture, leadership, communication, coordination, and problem solving/conflict management, was significantly related to lower risk-adjusted length of stay, lower nurse turnover, higher evaluated technical quality of care, and greater evaluated ability to meet family member needs. However, there was no significant effect of caregiver interaction on risk-adjusted mortality rates. There are several strengths of this study. First, it is theoretically driven, and its conceptual base is well described and documented. Second, the authors report appropriate information about instrument reliability and validity, including a brief discussion of the appropriateness of data aggregation. A concern noted is the small sample size ($N = 42$) and the low ratio of cases to variables (Thorndike, 1978).

McDaniel and Stumpf (1993) also used the OCI to measure aspects of culture from 250 randomly selected nurses in seven acute care hospitals in western Pennsylvania. The culture of the hospital was of interest here, in contrast to the work reported earlier of Coeling and Simms (1993a, 1993b), in which the culture of the nursing unit was the focus. Compared to the "ideal" nursing culture (as described by Thomas et al., 1990), McDaniel and Stumpf (1993) found the constructive culture was rated slightly lower and the aggressive/defensive and the passive/defensive cultures were rated slightly higher. McDaniel and Stumpf also found that the constructive culture was positively related to work satisfaction, overall satisfaction, retention (plans to stay in the organization for a year), and willingness of the nurse to recommend the organization to a friend as a place of employment.

The contribution of this study is that it is the first in nursing to attempt systematically to relate culture to other key organizational variables. The sampling plan, based on power analysis, was well described. Reliability coefficients for most of the scales used in the study were reported, but little detailed information about the validity of the scales was furnished. A surprising finding of this study was the lack of inter- and intrasite variance on the OCI among hospitals and nurses. This essentially means that the cultures of the different hospitals were perceived similarly and this similarity in perception extended to managers and staff nurses. The implications of this finding are not discussed by the authors, except perhaps peripherally when they acknowledge the limitations of the voluntary nature of the sample from a single geographic area. And although it is generally desirable to relate one's findings to earlier research, it is unclear why the authors were interested in comparing their findings with the ideal culture described by Thomas et al. (1990), when information regarding the construction of that "ideal" culture was lacking, thus calling into question its validity.

Research on Other Aspects of Culture

Defining culture as "an amalgam of symbols, language, assumptions and behaviors," Fleeger (1993) used both qualitative and quantitative methods to examine organizational ideology in three semiurban Oregon hospitals. Fleeger used Harrison's (1972) questionnaire, in which individuals' perceptions of the culture were assessed as power-centered, role-centered, task-centered, or person-centered. However, Harrison's work focused on what he called the organization's "character," not its culture. This is another example of a lack of conceptual clarity in terminology used in organizational culture research. Fleeger (1993) also used a "qualitative assessment inventory" but provided little additional descriptive information. The focus of this study was on whether the culture (ideology) on the selected nursing units was consonant with the culture (ideology) of the overall hospital and with the culture of other occupational groups. Two of the units were found to have cultures that were "consonant" with other occupational groups and with the overall organizational culture, but the third indicated dissonance between the unit and the organizational and other professional cultures. This dissonance was characterized by, for example, a mismatch between professional and organizational goals, a norm of competition, and "us versus them."

Fleeger's (1993) study is important because it examines a broad range of cultural issues, thus recognizing the complexity of the concept of culture. A particularly valuable contribution is the investigation of cultural consonance/dissonance and thus the acknowledgment that organizational culture is not monolithic but that organizations have multiple cultures. However, essential information was missing from the article. For example, "ideology" was never defined, nor was there an operational definition of "consonance" or "dissonance." No information was provided about the reliability and validity of the instruments. Details about the sampling plan were not included. Also lacking were descriptions of other "occupational" and "professional" groups and how data from these groups were gathered and analyzed. These omissions seriously undermine the value of the information presented.

Nystrom (1993) focused on the relationships between norms (the unwritten rules that tell members how they should and should not behave), values (beliefs about what outcomes should be desired), and the job satisfaction, organizational commitment, and performance of 41 managers and 36 executive secretaries in 13 health care organizations. Nystrom found that, for both managers and secretaries, "task norms" were significantly and positively related to both job satisfaction and organizational commitment. Similarly, what Nystrom labeled "pragmatic values" (i.e., those emphasizing achievement, skill, risk, and organizational efficiency) were also significantly and positively related, in both groups, to job satisfaction and organizational commitment.

Similar to the study by McDaniel and Stumpf (1993) described earlier, the contribution of Nystrom's (1993) work is the investigation of the relationship of two aspects of culture—in this case, norms and values—to important organizational outcomes. However, no rationale was provided with regard to the sampling strategy, raising once again the issue of representativeness. Although Nystrom provided reliability coefficients for the instruments used in the study, there was no accompanying discussion of validity.

Summary

This section has reviewed research articles on organizational culture from the nursing and health services literature. Without exception, all of the articles discussed in this chapter have characterized organizational culture from the functionalist perspective: conceptualizing culture as something the organization has. The underlying assumption is that a better understanding of organizational culture can be used by managers to improve organizational performance. None of the articles conceptualized culture as root variable. This is reflected in the lack of attention to the process issues underlying the formation, manifestation, transmission, and reformulation of organizational culture (e.g., see Barley, 1983; Hatch, 1993; Sackmann, 1992). The chapter now turns to a discussion of the conceptual and methodological issues that are apparent in this review.

CONCEPTUAL ISSUES IN RESEARCH ON ORGANIZATIONAL CULTURE

The primary conceptual issue that must be addressed in enhancing nursing research on organizational culture is the need to reflect, in both conceptual and operational definitions, that organizational culture is a complex multidimensional phenomenon that is expressed in many levels of the organization. For example, with the exception of Nystrom (1993), who examined both norms and values, the investigators previously cited focused on a single dimension of culture in each study: rules (Coeling & Wilcox, 1988, 1990), ideology (Fleeger, 1993), cultural types (McDaniel & Stumpf, 1993; Shortell et al., 1991; Thomas et al., 1990; Zimmerman et al., 1993), or norms (Coeling & Simms, 1993a, 1993b; Nystrom, 1993). Researchers approached culture as a relatively simple rather than complex phenomenon and as one that is uni- rather than multidimensional. In addition, the previously cited lack of definitional clarity with regard to the terms "rules" and "norms" also calls attention to the need for additional conceptual precision. Fleeger's (1993) work on cultural consonance recognized the need to address the multilevel aspect of organizational culture by including assessments, not only of the nursing unit but of the overall culture as well. Notwithstanding the difficulties of doing research on organizational culture, nursing researchers would do well to remember Pettigrew's (1979) statement that culture should be considered a "family" of concepts— symbol, language, ideology, belief, ritual, and myth—as they conceptualize and design studies.

If the Reichers and Schneider (1990) stages in the evolution of concept development are used to evaluate research in organizational culture, it appears that the nursing and health services research on organizational culture still dwells in the first phase, that of introduction and elaboration. The articles were concerned primarily with simplified conceptualizations of culture. Some of the researchers began to examine the relationship between organizational culture and the change process (Coeling & Simms, 1993a, 1993b) or other key organizational variables (McDaniel & Stumpf, 1993; Nystrom, 1993; Shortell et al., 1993; Zimmerman et al., 1993, 1994), without placing the concept of culture in a broader, more encompassing theoretical framework. To date, no critical reviews of organizational culture research—a hallmark of the second phase, evaluation and augmentation—have appeared in either the nursing or health services research literature. Nor have the conditions of the third stage, consolidation and accommodation, appeared: the development of consensus on conceptualization and operationalization as well as on antecedents, consequences, and boundary conditions. Culture has been examined from a pragmatic rather than a theoretical perspective. Consequently, knowledge development regarding a "theory of culture" in either nursing or in health services is lacking.

METHODOLOGICAL ISSUES

This section is divided into two parts. The first part summarizes the critiques with regard to (a) conceptual and operational definitions of organizational culture, (b) adequacy of sampling plans, and, (c) information about the psychometric properties of the research instruments. In contrast to the previous section, which commented on conceptual issues in the study of organizational culture, this section focuses specifically on the methodological implications of a lack of consistency between conceptual and operational definitions of organizational culture. Perhaps because of small samples, authors have relied primarily on simple, descriptive statistical analyses; the analyses are therefore not reviewed here. The exception was Shortell et al. (1994), who used regression analysis. The second part of this section discusses the appropriate treatment of the "unit of analysis" in organizational culture research.

Summary of Critiques

Little of the research reported in this review has been published in research journals; seven of the articles were published in nursing journals whose primary audience is practitioners. Of these, six were published in the *Journal of Nursing Administration* (Coeling & Simms, 1993a, 1993b; Coeling & Wilcox, 1988; delBueno & Vincent, 1986; McDaniel & Stumpf, 1993; Thomas et al., 1990); the seventh article (Coeling & Wilcox, 1990) was published in a clinically oriented nursing journal. Another article was published in a health care management journal that has primarily a practitioner readership (Nystrom, 1993). Only four articles (Shortell et al., 1991, 1994; Zimmerman et al., 1993, 1994) were published in research-oriented journals. Consequently, it is difficult to evaluate accurately the quality of the research, and this critique should be understood in that context.

Conceptual and Operational Definitions.   Possibly because the conceptual construal of organizational culture is so complex and multidimensional and its boundaries so indeterminate, researchers can choose from a vast assortment of conceptual definitions. This diversity in conceptual definitions is apparent in the articles reviewed here, despite the small number. Coeling and Wilcox (1988, 1990) defined organizational culture as a "set of solutions devised by a group of people to meet specific problems posed by the situations they face in common" (1988, p. 16; 1990, p. 231). Thomas et al. (1990) and McDaniel and Stumpf (1993) defined culture as "the ways of thinking, behaving, and believing that members of a unit have in common." Shortell et al. (1991) defined culture similarly, as "the norms, values, beliefs and expectations shared by people who work in a given unit" (p. 710). In these instances the authors' operational definitions were consistent with their conceptual definitions, providing some evidence of face validity. In contrast, Fleeger (1993) defined culture as an "amalgam of symbols, language, assumptions and behaviors" (p. 39) but operationally examined ideology without articulating the logical or theoretical linkages between the construct and the selected empirical indicators. Nystrom's report (1993) exhibited a similar problem: without providing a specific conceptual definition of organizational culture, Nystrom focused operationally on norms (i.e., "the unwritten rules that tell members how they should and should not behave" [p. 43]) and values (i.e., "beliefs about what outcomes should be desired or preferred" [p. 43]). This lack of correspondence between a concept and its empirical indicators significantly reduces construct validity and contributes to difficulty in building a solid body of knowledge about the concept under investigation.

Sampling Strategies.   Sampling strategies were rarely described in adequate detail. Of the quantitative studies reviewed here, only McDaniel and Stumpf (1993) used probability sampling based on power analysis. Shortell et al. (1991, 1994) used a two-stage sampling plan with a national sample of 42 ICUs, of which 26 were randomly selected. Within each ICU, a convenience sample of individuals was used. Zimmerman et al. (1993) purposively selected 9 ICUs from the 42 ICUs included in the Shortell et al. (1993) study. The more frequent occurrence was a simple statement of how many subjects participated (Coeling & Simms, 1993b; Nystrom, 1993; Thomas et al., 1990). In one case (Fleeger, 1993), other than the fact that individuals in three hospitals participated in the research, no other information about respondents was furnished. Even in the qualitative studies there was inadequate information about the underlying rationale that guided sample selection (Coeling & Wilcox, 1988, 1990). In research on organizational culture, whether quantitative or qualitative, a variety of sampling plans (probability or nonprobability) may be appropriate. It remains incumbent upon the authors of published reports, however, to explain the rationale for sample selection.

Psychometric Properties of Research Instruments.   Few of the articles reviewed here provided full information on reliability and validity. McDaniel and Stumpf (1993) and Nystrom (1993) reported information on reliability (alpha coefficients), but information on validity is either insufficient (McDaniel & Stumpf, 1993) or completely lacking (Nystrom, 1993). The Shortell et al. (1994) article provided appropriate information on reliability and validity for their perceptual measures. In an article whose purpose it was to describe the use of the OCI, Thomas et al. (1990) did not report any information about instrument psychometrics. Although Coeling and Simms (1993a, 1993b) went into some detail about the development of the NUCAT, the articles did not provide adequate information for a reader to thoroughly evaluate the instrument.

Once again, it must be recognized that the journals in which the vast majority of these articles were published were not research journals. The critical methodological details, to which the authors may have given appropriate attention in their research, possibly were edited out from the published article.

Unit of Analysis in Organizational Culture Research

An important methodological issue that needs to be more fully recognized in quantitative research on organizational culture, when culture is treated as a variable, rather than as a root metaphor, is the appropriate definition and treatment of the "unit of analysis." Organizational culture can be conceptualized as either a psychological variable, in which case it is measured at the individual level; organizational culture can also be conceptualized as a group or organizational level variable, in which case data are generally collected from individuals and the data then aggregated to the higher (i.e., group or organizational) level. Aggregation refers to the process of combining information from one level, in this case the individual level, to represent attributes of a higher level, in this case, the nursing unit or the organization (James, 1982). In individual level research, the sample size is the number of individual respondents/participants, while in aggregate level research, the sample size is the number of aggregated units.

Perceptual agreement on aggregated scale scores, in this case, scores, for example on the OCI or the NUCAT, indicate the extent to which there is sufficient agreement about organizational culture within the specified group (i.e., the nursing unit) to use a mean score to represent that group. A small amount of "within-group" variance relative to "between-group" variance suggests that the aggregated score (i.e., mean) is appropriate to represent the group (James, 1982). Similarly, when differences between groups are large, one assumes higher levels of agreement, whereas when differences within groups are large, one assumes a lower level of agreement. The literature is replete with a variety of statistical methods (and a fair amount of controversy) with which to assess the level of perceptual agreement: analysis of variance, indices of interrater reliability in a single group (Glick, 1985), eta squared (Dansereau & Alutto, 1990; Shortell et al., 1991) and correlations among the perceptions of individuals occupying various organizational levels (Jones & James, 1979).

Most of the quantitative studies reviewed here treated organizational culture as an individual level phenomenon (Fleeger, 1993; McDaniel & Stumpf, 1993; Nystrom, 1993; Thomas et al., 1990), whereas Coeling and Simms (1993a, 1993b), Shortell et al. (1991, 1994), and Zimmerman et al. (1993) treated culture as a group level phenomenon. Only Shortell et al. (1991, 1994), however, furnished a discussion about their evaluation of the appropriateness of using the aggregated mean score. With regard to sample size, it is difficult to ascertain from the Coeling and Simms (1993a, 1993b) articles whether they considered their sample size to be the 33 nursing units or the 607 individuals who participated. Conceptualizing culture as a group level phenomenon suggests that the appropriate sample size is 33. In contrast, in the Shortell et al. (1991, 1994) articles, it is clear that the sample size is the number of intensive care units (42), not the individual number of participants.

Similarly, when data are aggregated from the individual to the group level, instrument psychometrics must be evaluated at the group, rather than at the individual level (Glick, 1985; Sirotnick, 1980; Verran, Mark, & Lamb, 1992). Estimates of the reliability of aggregated data may be calculated through the use of interitem-correlations among raters, mean rater reliability based on items and mean rater reliability based on scale scores, in which case, an intraclass correlation coefficient (ICC) is used (Glick, 1985; James, 1982). Glick (1985) suggested that each of these estimates should be greater than .60 to support the use of aggregated measures. However, researchers should also be aware of the assumptions underlying use of the ICC: a large random sample of organizations, random selection of raters, homogeneity of variance within organizations, and equal numbers of raters in each organization. Only the two articles by Shortell et al. (1991, 1994) addressed these issues.

DIRECTIONS FOR FUTURE RESEARCH

By and large, the research described in this review has focused on simple conceptualizations of culture. Yet organizational culture is a much richer phenomenon than simply the rules and norms or ideologies of an organization. Even if one does elect to examine rules or norms, the processes by which these rules or norms are transmitted to organization members has not been explored, nor has anyone described the processes by which rules or norms change over time. Does culture reside in the "workers" or can it, as is implied in many popular management articles, be changed by a conscious effort of top management?

None of the articles reported here examined culture from the interpretivist perspective (e.g., the symbolic nature of culture or of culture as process), two enormously rich areas for further exploration. How, for example, do cultural artifacts become symbols, that is, gain meaning beyond their "literal domain"? How do these symbols then serve to maintain the organization's culture? How does an individual "learn" the culture in the organization? What is the process by which culture is internalized? Is that process cognitive, linguistic, behavioral, or emotional, or do some individuals rely primarily on one rather than another type of process? At what point in the process of internalization does the individual become cognizant of behaving in culturally acceptable ways? And where in that process might the individual (or group) prove to be the most amenable to change?

The questions raised above suggest some avenues for further research on organizational culture. Underlying these questions is a call to recognize in our research the subtle and multifaceted nature of organizational culture, to design research (whether qualitative or quantitative) that is methodologically sound, and to publish sufficient information that allows a more comprehensive critical appraisal of the research.

ACKNOWLEDGMENT

The assistance of Vicki Fisher, MS, RN, and Charlotte McDaniel, PhD, RN, in the preparation of this article is acknowleged.

NOTES

1. This chapter will explore a variety of definitions of organizational culture. Whatever one's definition, however, organizational culture is conceptually distinct from organizational climate, which reflects "perceptions of organizational structures and how it *feels* to be a member of the organization" (Cooke & Rousseau, 1988, p. 251).

2. Although this article did not meet the inclusion criteria as previously outlined, it is briefly discussed because of its contribution to understanding the subsequent development of the nursing literature on organizational culture.

REFERENCES

Barley, S. (1983). Semiotics and the study of occupational and organizational cultures. *Administrative Science Quarterly, 28*, 393–413.

Coeling, H., & Simms, L. (1993a). Facilitating innovation at the nursing unit level through cultural assessment: Part 1. *Journal of Nursing Administration, 23*(4), 46–53.

Coeling, H., & Simms, L. (1993b). Facilitating innovation at the nursing unit level through cultural assessment: Part 2. *Journal of Nursing Administration, 23*(5), 13–20.

Coeling, H., & Wilcox, J. (1988). Understanding organizational culture. *Journal of Nursing Administration, 18*(11), 16–22.

Coeling, H., & Wilcox, J. (1990). Using organizational culture to facilitate the change process. *ANNA Journal, 17*, 231–236.

Cooke, R., & Lafferty, J. (1989). Organizational culture inventory. Plymouth, MI: Human Synergistics.

Cooke, R., & Rousseau, D. (1988). Behavioral norms and expectations. *Group and Organizational Studies, 13*, 245–273.

Dansereau, F., & Alutto, J. (1990). Level-of-analysis issues in climate and culture research. In B. Schneider (Ed.), *Organizational climate and culture* (pp. 193–236). San Francisco: Jossey-Bass.

del Bueno, D. J., & Vincent, P. M. (1986). Organizational culture: How important is it? *Journal of Nursing Administration, 16*(10), 15–20.

Fleeger, M. E. (1993). Assessing organizational culture: A planning strategy. *Nursing Management, 24*(2), 39–41.

Glick, W. (1985). Conceptualizing and measuring organizational and psychological climate: Pitfalls in multilevel research. *Academy of Management Review, 10*, 601–616.

Harrison, R. (1972). Understanding your organization's character. *Harvard Business Review, 50*(3), 119–128.

Hatch, M. (1993). The dynamics of organizational culture. *Academy of Management Review, 18*, 657–693.

James, L. (1982). Aggregation bias in estimates of perceptual agreement. *Journal of Applied Psychology, 67*, 219–229.

Jones, A., & James, L. (1979). Psychological climate: Dimensions and relationships of individual and aggregated work environment perceptions. *Organizational Behavior and Human Performance, 23*, 201–250.

McDaniel, C., & Stumpf, L. (1993). The organizational culture: Implications for nursing service. *Journal of Nursing Administration, 23*(4), 54–60.

Mumby, D. (1994). Review of the book *Culture in organizations. Three perspectives. Academy of Management Review, 19*(1), 156–159.

Nystrom, P. (1993). Organizational cultures, strategies and commitments in health care organizations. *Health Care Management Review, 18*, 43–49.

Pettigrew, A. (1979). On studying organizational cultures. *Administrative Science Quarterly, 24*, 570–580.

Reichers, A., & Schneider, B. (1990). Climate and culture: An evolution of concepts. In B. Schneider (Ed.), *Organizational climate and culture* (pp. 5–39). San Francisco: Jossey-Bass.

Sackmann, S. (1992). Culture and subcultures: An analysis of organizational knowledge. *Administrative Science Quarterly, 37*, 140–161.

Shortell, S., Rousseau, D., Gillies, R., Devers, K., & Simons, B. (1991). Organizational assessment in intensive care units (ICUs): Construct development, reliability, and validity of the ICU nurse-physician questionnaire. *Medical Care, 29*, 709–726.

Shortell, S., Zimmerman, J., Rousseau, D., Gillies, R., Wagner, D., Draper, E., Knaus, W., & Duffy, J. (1994). The performance of intensive care units: Does good management make a difference? *Medical Care, 32*, 508–525.

Sirotnick, K. (1980). Psychometric implications of the unit-of-analysis problem (with examples from the measurement of organizational climate). *Journal of Educational Measurement, 17*, 245–282.

Smircich, L. (1983). Concepts of culture and organizational analysis. *Administrative Science Quarterly, 28*, 339–358.

Smircich, L. (1985). Is the concept of culture a paradigm for understanding organizations and ourselves? In P. Frost, L. Moore, M. Louis, C. Lundberg, & J. Martin, (Eds), *Organizational culture* (pp. 55–72). Beverly Hills: Sage.

Thomas, C., Ward, M., Chorba, C., & Kumiega, A. (1990). Measuring and interpreting organizational culture. *Journal of Nursing Administration, 20*(6), 17–24.

Thorndike, R. (1978). *Correlational procedures for research.* New York: Gardner Press.

Verran, J., Mark, B., & Lamb, G. (1992) Psychometric examination of instruments using aggregated data. *Research in Nursing and Health, 15*, 237–240.

Wilkins, A. (1983). The culture audit: A tool for understanding organizations. *Organizational Dynamics, 12*, 24–38.

Zimmerman, J., Rousseau, D., Duffy, J., Devers, K., Gillies, R., Wagner, D., Draper, E., Shortell, S., & Knaus, W. (1994). Intensive care at two teaching hospitals: An organizational case study. *American Journal of Critical Care, 3*, 129–138.

Zimmerman, J., Shortell, S., Rousseau, D., Duffy, J., Gillies, R., Knaus, W., Devers, K., Wagner, D., & Draper, E. (1993). Improving intensive care: Observations based on organizational case studies in nine intensive care units: A prospective, multicenter study. *Critical Care Medicine, 21*, 1443–1451.

PART III
Research on Nursing Education

Chapter 8

Oncology Nursing Education

M. LINDA WORKMAN
FRANCES PAYNE BOLTON SCHOOL OF NURSING
CASE WESTERN RESERVE UNIVERSITY

CONTENTS

Cancer has been and remains a major health problem afflicting millions of people worldwide. With advances in treatment, cancer as a disease has changed from being an acute and terminal condition to being a chronic condition with periods of acute problems. Optimal health care for people with cancer, whether the intent of the care is curative or supportive, requires specialized knowledge and skills delivered by nurses who understand the person's position within the cancer experience.

Although cancer is an old problem, the specialty of oncology nursing is of relatively recent origin. Interest in this specialization closely parallels the advancing technologies that have led to an increase both in cancer cure rates and in overall survival time. This chapter is focused on the research guiding the process of development in oncology nursing education during the past several decades.

Data for this review were collected through the use of computerized literature searches (SilverPlatter, MEDLINE). Other methods used to identify relevant studies included retrieval of archival materials from organizations related to cancer and oncology nursing, such as Oncology Nursing Society and American Cancer Society, and interviews with professionals responsible for the development of oncology nursing as a practice specialty, particularly the American Cancer Society Professors of Oncology Nursing and the Education Committee of the Oncology Nursing Society. Research methods used in identification of problems related to oncology nursing development and education focused primarily on information derived from national surveys, delphi studies, and consensus groups. Studies evaluating the educational programs or interventions used surveys, group case reports, and data obtained through certification testing.

Information presented in this review of research in oncology nursing education is divided into the following three sections: (a) research related to undergraduate curricula in cancer and oncology nursing, (b) research related to graduate nursing curricula in cancer and oncology nursing, and (c) research related to continuing education in cancer and oncology nursing.

UNDERGRADUATE ONCOLOGY NURSING EDUCATION

The prevalence of cancer as a common health problem, with one in three Americans expected to develop cancer at some point, leads one to expect that information regarding cancer development, prevention, early detection, treatment, and nursing care needs would constitute a major focus of basic undergraduate nursing education. However, research revealed that the topic of cancer in basic nursing programs has not and does not currently receive time and attention in proportion to the percentage of patients with cancer that nursing students and graduate nurses are likely to encounter in everyday nursing practice.

The Past

The dearth of oncology nursing education within basic programs was first identified by Diller (1955), who surveyed the cancer content of the curricula of 91 selected schools of nursing during the 1950s (Craytor, 1982; Diller, 1955). On the basis of the results obtained, Diller proposed a plan to integrate cancer concepts into undergraduate nursing education at the baccalaureate level. Her proposal was funded by the National Cancer Institute and first implemented at Skidmore College. Four additional baccalaureate programs in nursing, at Boston University, University of California at Los Angeles, Vanderbilt University, and Washington University at St. Louis, also were funded at this time to increase cancer-related content within the curriculum (Hilkemeyer, 1982; Peterson, 1956). Diller, an expert in education research, also developed a tool to measure cancer knowledge among nursing students. This tool formed the basis of evaluation for the effectiveness of the National Cancer Institute program that integrated cancer concepts into baccalaureate nursing education.

The formal integration of cancer content into baccalaureate nursing programs remained the exception rather than the rule from the 1950s through the 1970s. A major impetus for change was initiated by nurses involved in the service side of nursing rather than the education side. Hospital-based nursing supervisors and head nurses were faced with graduate nurses who lacked even basic knowledge about the care of people with cancer. Medical and nursing staffs at large cancer treatment centers, together with units of the American Cancer Society, developed cancer nursing workshops for new graduates and nursing students. Where such workshops existed, they became a popular means of exposing nursing students to accurate information regarding cancer prevention, development, treatment, and nursing care, without forcing the participation of nurse educators (Craytor, 1982).

Until the 1970s, undergraduate nursing curricula only indirectly addressed the topics of cancer and oncology nursing. Students were assigned to provide nursing care to patients with cancer, but cancer content generally was not included in medical-surgical nursing classes (Hilkemeyer, 1982). When cancer content was presented, often by a physician, the focus was on pathology and treatment outcomes rather than on nursing needs and supportive care. Often the only formal discussion of cancer-related issues in nursing education occurred within the context of pediatric nursing education (Hilkemeyer, 1982).

Brown, Johnson, and Groenwald (1983) conducted a national survey of all schools of nursing accredited by the National League for Nursing (NLN) to determine the total amount of time devoted to topics relevant to oncology nursing within basic undergraduate nursing curricula. The survey response rate was 75%, and the educational level of the responding schools was representative of the national breakdown of the NLN-accredited programs. Although their results showed considerable variation in the amount of educational time spent in disseminating oncology nursing content (a total mean of 14.5 hours per student per school), few schools adequately or accurately covered identified essential content.

The Present

The Education Committee of the Oncology Nursing Society and the professional education committees of various units and divisions of the American Cancer Society have conducted many regional and national surveys of cancer content in basic nursing programs up to the present (Belani & Belcher, 1994;

Frerichs & Varricchio, 1988; Quinn-Casper & Holmgren, 1987). The findings of these recent surveys continue to support the earlier findings that core knowledge about oncology nursing in basic programs is inadequate and often inaccurate. In addition, the surveys also indicated that students in general have a poor attitude toward oncology nursing. Students view oncology nursing as depressing, futile, behind the times in a high-technology profession, and unimportant.

In many instances the poor attitudes of nursing students toward oncology nursing also reflected those of the faculty responsible for implementation of cancer content. Moreover, surveys indicated that many faculty teaching core content in oncology nursing had inadequate backgrounds for this specialty (Belcher, 1987; Brown et al., 1982; Diller, 1955; Frerichs & Varricchio, 1988). Thus, information disseminated in class was not only scant, it was often inaccurate or outdated.

Although core content in oncology nursing education in most basic nursing programs has been demonstrated to be inadequate, electives in oncology nursing are beginning to fill the gap on a limited scale. Most basic nursing programs that have one or more elective educational experiences in oncology nursing are at large universities associated with major cancer treatment centers and have significant interaction with the American Cancer Society or the Oncology Nursing Society. Usually, the faculty member coordinating the elective experience either has a specialty in oncology at the master's level or oncology nursing clinical experience or has received continuing education preparation in issues related to cancer and oncology nursing. Such elective experiences include in-depth oncology courses (Horvitz & Trigg, 1986; Nevidjon & Deatrich, 1985), extracurricular sponsored workshops (Quinn-Casper & Holmgren, 1987), independent studies (Belcher, 1987; Mooney & Dudas, 1987), and preceptor-guided focused clinical experiences (Oishi, Oki, Itano, Stringfellow, & Kurren, 1986).

Studies on the effectiveness of such programs show positive changes in the areas of knowledge and attitudes among participating students. In general, the faculty providing or coordinating the experiences have greater knowledge and more positive attitudes regarding oncology nursing than do faculty at basic nursing education programs where oncology elective experiences do not exist. However, because the in-depth oncology nursing courses tend to be elective in nature, the existence of such courses does little to fill the gaps in basic nursing education related to cancer and oncology nursing.

Currently, some strides are being made at regional levels to correct the problems of lack of interest in the topic and inadequate knowledge levels among the faculty responsible for teaching the oncology nursing content in undergraduate nursing programs. In some instances, American Cancer Society divisions are taking the lead in "Educate the Educator" or "Train the Trainer" programs. These programs offer audiovisual and resource support to the faculty being trained as well as providing them with the means to acquire an adequate knowledge base in oncology nursing (Palos, personal communication, May 1991). In other situations, oncology nurses are serving as faculty, providing classroom information regarding cancer and oncology nursing. Such programs have been successful on a local or regional scale. Their feasibility on a broader scale has yet to be determined.

In 1992 the Oncology Nursing Society conducted a follow-up survey of all NLN-accredited schools of nursing to again determine the time and type of educational methods used to teach essential oncology content in basic nursing education programs. Data analysis from this survey is not yet completed. Results of this survey can be used to evaluate different educational strategies for teaching essential oncology nursing content to undergraduate nursing students.

GRADUATE ONCOLOGY NURSING EDUCATION

The Oncology Nursing Society and the American Cancer Society have taken the position that oncology nursing care is optimal when managed or at least overseen by advanced practice nurses, either clinical specialists or nurse practitioners, who have master's degrees with a major in oncology nursing (American Cancer Society & Oncology Nursing Society, 1988). Content requirements for such programs are based on the *Standards of Oncology Nursing Education* developed for the advanced practice level by the Oncology Nursing Society (1989). The intended outcomes of these standards are to (a) enhance the quality of oncology nursing education and (b) improve health care for the public. Research reports indicated that development of the standards of practice and the educational requirements for the advanced practice level of oncology nursing was based on empirically derived data (American Cancer Society & Oncology Nursing Society, 1979; Hennessey & Wright, 1980; McGee, Powell, Broadwell, & Clark, 1987; Siehl, 1982; Spross, 1983).

The Past

The first graduate program with an emphasis on oncology nursing was established in 1947 at Teacher's College, Columbia University (Craytor, 1982; Hilkemeyer, 1982; Piemme, 1985). This course of study was part of a program leading to a master's degree. The first graduate nursing program leading to a master's degree in science in nursing, with a major in oncology nursing, was established at the University of Pittsburgh in 1968. Both of these programs were developed with assistance from the American Cancer Society. Additional graduate oncology nursing programs were implemented as the clinical nurse specialist role in advanced nursing practice became more accepted (Benner, 1985; Given, 1980; Henke, 1980; Mauksch, 1989).

By 1980 more than a dozen graduate nursing programs offered specialization in oncology nursing. There was considerable variation in the actual content of these different programs. The oncology nursing education experts from the American Cancer Society, together with members of the relatively new Oncology Nursing Society, began consensus building in 1978 in an effort to establish a common essential role for the oncology clinical specialist and to develop an appropriate graduate oncology nursing curriculum (American Cancer Society & Oncology Nursing Society, 1979; Craytor, 1982). Recommendations for graduate oncology program planning and implementation were published in 1979. These recommendations were updated in 1988 (American Cancer Society & Oncology Nursing Society, 1988) as a result of information obtained through modified delphi surveys, expert panel consensus groups, and surveys of practicing oncology clinical nurse specialists (Hamric, 1985; McGee et al., 1987; Paulen, 1985, Siehl, 1982; Spross, 1983; Spross & Donoghue, 1984; Welch-McCaffrey, 1986; Yasko, 1983).

Although a common graduate oncology nursing curriculum was recommended and master's degree programs usually included all components of the recommended content, variation in program emphasis was apparent. One explanation for variation in emphasis rested with the interests and expertise of the faculty members responsible for the program. For example, pediatric oncology was a major focus for graduate oncology programs having faculty members who were experts in pediatric oncology. Psychosocial issues were given priority over other practice issues in programs in which the expertise or research interests of the faculty were more psychosocial than physiological.

The Present

The number of graduate oncology nursing programs has continued to increase incrementally during the past decade ("Assessing Graduate Education," 1980; Brown & Hinds, 1993; McGee, 1988; McMillan, 1988). The 1993 survey (Brown & Hinds, 1993) of colleges and universities in the United States showed 42 graduate oncology nursing programs in 26 states and the District of Columbia. This survey indicated continued variation in specialization content over and above recommended content.

At a time when many master's specialization programs are experiencing an enrollment drop-off, enthusiasm for advanced practice in oncology nursing continues, and enrollment in graduate oncology nursing programs remains relatively steady (Brown & Hinds, 1993). Maintenance of enrollment may be related to the continued nationwide need for advanced practice nurses with specialization in oncology and to the availability of scholarship support. Financial support for students engaging in graduate oncology nursing education is available through several funding agencies. The American Cancer Society has provided substantial support for over 200 graduate students in oncology nursing since the inception of the American Cancer Society Scholarship Program in 1981 (Fernsler & Holcombe, 1994; Frerichs & Yasko, 1985). The Oncology Nursing Society also funds scholarships for graduate education in oncology nursing.

Some schools of nursing maintain the traditional clinical nurse specialist as the product, and other schools of nursing have expanded the scope of the curriculum to include the oncology nurse practitioner as the product. Many different strategies to achieve the goals of graduate oncology nursing curricula have been implemented, including the use of clinical nurse specialists as preceptors, mentorship programs, and the use of longitudinal caseloads (Fenton, 1992; Hagopian, Ferszt, Jacobs, & McCorkle, 1992; Moore, Piper, Dodd, & Hudes, 1987). Program evaluation research is ongoing and largely presents graduates and individual programs as case reports (Hamric, 1985; McMillan, 1987; Moore et al., 1987). The American Cancer Society Professors of Oncology Nursing, together with members of the Education Committee of the Oncology Nursing Society, are revising the pamphlet titled *The Master's Degree with a Specialty in Oncology Nursing* to include essential oncology nursing content for oncology nurse practitioners as well as for oncology clinical nurse specialists.

CONTINUING ONCOLOGY NURSING EDUCATION

Most people with cancer receive nursing care at the hands of generalists rather than specialists in oncology nursing. Therefore, oncology nursing education experts associated with the Oncology Nursing Society and the American Cancer Society first defined oncology nursing education at the fundamental level and the advanced level (Given, 1980). The fundamental level, now known as the generalist level, is defined as "the level of practice for a registered nurse who possesses general knowledge and skills applicable to diversified health concerns of clients" (Oncology Nursing Society, 1989, p. 17). Although such a definition is broad enough to include all registered nurses who participate on any level in the care of people with cancer, the application of the definition is focused on those who routinely provide some aspect of nursing care to people with cancer.

The Past

As discussed earlier in this chapter, undergraduate nursing education related to cancer and oncology nursing in the United States has long been identified as inadequate. This inadequacy was first identified by nursing supervisors and head nurses of new nursing graduates, "generalists" who were expected to provide basic nursing care to patients with cancer. The literature abounds with articles documenting the educational needs of practicing generalist registered nurses providing care to patients with cancer ("C-COP Program," 1983; Craytor, 1982; Craytor, Brown & Morrow, 1978; Donaldson et al., 1988; Hennesey & Wright, 1980; Piper, 1981).

The recognition that oncology was a rapidly changing field and that generalist nurses taking care of cancer patients needed a means to keep pace with knowledge and technological advances had several major outcomes. The first was the development of government-funded formal programs targeted to nurses working in community hospitals, where access to cancer-related courses, workshops, and continuing education programs was limited. These programs included the Cancer Centers Outreach Program (C-COP) and the Clinical Hospital Oncology Program (CHOP) ("C-COP Program," 1983; Hilkemeyer, 1982). The focus of such programs was to improve the quality of care provided to cancer patients through clinician education and the availability of standard treatment protocols for specific cancers.

A second outcome was the establishment of the Oncology Nursing Society in 1975 as a national specialty nursing organization (Craytor, 1982; Hilkemeyer, 1982; Reed-Ash, 1988). Prior to the establishment of the national Oncology Nursing Society, small local groups of oncology nurses banded together and attempted to meet their own learning needs. The ultimate purpose in founding the Oncology Nursing Society was to put forth a unified effort in providing educational support to nurses involved in any aspect of the care of patients with cancer. This task involved the development of standards of practice for the generalist level and the building of programs to assist nurses in meeting those standards (Blausey, Barton, & Dicke, 1984; Clark & McGee, 1992; Howell, 1986; Oncology Nursing Society, 1989).

The Present

Workshops and continuing education programs incorporating oncology nursing content represent a substantial portion of continuing nursing education. The American Cancer Society and the Oncology Nursing Society remain proactive forces, putting forth high-quality programs to meet the continuing education needs of generalist nurses involved in oncology nursing. The Oncology Nursing Society continues to survey its over 20,000 members for educational needs (Fernsler, 1987; Itano & Miller, 1990). Programs are tailored to meet the needs of nurses working in community settings (Krohner & Spitak, 1992) and rural settings (Bushy & Kost, 1990). Recently, the programs were expanded to those providing care to minority populations (Palos, personal communication, May 1991).

CONCLUSIONS

The research literature focused on oncology nursing education indicated that the recommended educational strategies in use currently are based on information obtained from a broad educational data base. However, most of the data have an academic or curriculum content focus. No reports were available regarding the relationship between basic and graduate oncology nursing content presented in formal nursing programs and the quality of care for patients and families experiencing cancer.

Development of research in oncology nursing education has been the responsibility of the Education Committee of the Oncology Nursing Society and professional education programs (both statewide and national) of the American Cancer Society. The greatest number of research efforts have been made in graduate education and in continuing education in oncology nursing. Undergraduate oncology nursing education remains the area with the least consistency in educational strategies and has greatest need for change.

The identified weaknesses in undergraduate oncology nursing education appear to have two origins: faculty attitudes and emphasis on the generalist role. Historically, faculty attitudes toward cancer and oncology nursing have been negative. Such attitudes are reflected in the planning and implementation of curricula. When cancer and oncology nursing are presented as "futile" and "depressing" because many patients eventually succumb to the disease, the focus of nursing as a science and art of caring rather than curing is debased. In addition, the position that undergraduate education must "cover the waterfront" in all areas of health and illness so that students will be successful on the National Council Licensure Examination for Registered Nurses (NCLEX-RN) exams dilutes the level of importance placed on oncology nursing education.

RECOMMENDATIONS FOR FUTURE RESEARCH

Ongoing research in oncology nursing education is necessary to improve the quality of care that all patients with cancer receive. The area of greatest need is undergraduate oncology nursing education. Research has led to the identification of problem areas and to the development and implementation of a few strategies for ameliorating the identified problems. Further research is needed to evaluate the impact of the intervention strategies and to develop additional interventions.

One area possibly amenable to research is the NCLEX-RN. Undergraduate nursing curricula frequently are driven by the pressure to have students perform well on the licensing examination. As a result, curricula are developed to "teach to" the NCLEX-RN. Research into how much of the NCLEX-RN is devoted to issues related to oncology nursing, in addition to how well students perform overall on oncology nursing test items, could provide the impetus for curriculum revision.

A major issue for advanced practice is certification. Currently, oncology nursing certification remains at the generalist level. The Oncology Nursing Society is in the process of working with the American Nurses Association to develop an advanced practice certification. Future research should be focused on the impact of advanced practice certification on graduate oncology nursing education, patient education regarding cancer prevention and early detection, and the quality of nursing care that people with cancer receive.

REFERENCES

American Cancer Society & Oncology Nursing Society. (1979). *The master's degree with a specialty in oncology nursing.* Pittsburgh, PA: Oncology Nursing Society.

American Cancer Society & Oncology Nursing Society. (1988). *The master's degree with a specialty in oncology nursing.* Pittsburgh, PA: Oncology Nursing Society.

Assessing graduate education in oncology nursing. (1980). *Oncology Nursing Forum, 7*(1), 37–38.

Belani, C., & Belcher, A. (1994). Instruction in the techniques and concept of supportive care in oncology. *Supportive Care and Cancer, 2,* 50–55.

Belcher, A. (1987). Defining content and methods. *Oncology Nursing Forum, 14*(5), 65–67.

Benner, P. (1985). The oncology clinical nurse specialist: An expert coach. *Oncology Nursing Forum, 12*(2), 40–44.

Blausey, L., Barton, P., & Dicke, R. (1984). Development of nursing care guidelines: Putting the ONS outcome standards to work. *Oncology Nursing Forum, 11*(1), 54–58.

Brown, J., & Hinds, P. (1993). Assessing master's programs in oncology nursing. *Oncology Nursing Forum, 20,* 1425–1433.

Brown, J., Johnson, J., & Groenwald, S. (1983). Survey of cancer nursing education in US schools of nursing. *Oncology Nursing Forum, 10*(4), 82–83.

Bushy, A., & Kost, S. (1990). A model of continuing education for rural oncology nurses. *Oncology Nursing Forum, 17,* 207–211.

C-COP Program funded (cross country). (1983). *Oncology Nursing Forum, 10*(4), 112.

Clark, J., & McGee, R. (Eds). (1992). *Core curriculum for oncology nursing* (2nd ed.). Philadelphia: Saunders.

Craytor, J. (1982). Highlights in education for cancer nursing. *Oncology Nursing Forum, 9*(4), 51–59.

Craytor, J., Brown, J., & Morrow, G. (1978). Assessing learning needs of nurses who care for persons with cancer. *Cancer Nursing, 1*, 211–220.

Diller, D. (1955). *An investigation of cancer learning in ninety-one selected schools of nursing.* Saratoga Springs, NY: Skidmore College Press.

Donaldson, W., Glass, E., Helmick, F., Ezzone, S., Kellerstraus, B., & Stevenson, B. (1988). Determining continuing education priorities in cancer management for nurses. *Oncology Nursing Forum, 15*, 625–630.

Fenton, M. (1992). Education for the advanced practice of clinical nurse specialists. *Oncology Nursing Forum, 19*(Suppl.), 16–20.

Fernsler, J. (1987). Developing continuing education programs in cancer nursing: An overview. *Oncology Nursing Forum, 14*(5), 59–60.

Fernsler, J., & Holcombe, J. (1994). A survey of recipients of American Cancer Society master's degree scholarships. *Oncology Nursing Forum, 21*, 763–767.

Frerichs, M., & Varricchio, C. (1988). An assessment of student nurses' knowledge about cancer. *Oncology Nursing Forum, 15*, 631–633.

Frerichs, M., & Yasko, J. (1985). The American Cancer Society's scholarship program. *Oncology Nursing Forum, 12*(1), 62–64.

Given, B. (1980). Education of the oncology nurse: The key to excellent patient care. *Seminars in Oncology, 7*(1), 71–79.

Hagopian, G., Ferszt, G., Jacobs, L., & McCorkle, R. (1992). Preparing clinical preceptors to teach master's-level students in oncology nursing. *Journal of Professional Nursing, 8*, 295–300.

Hamric, A. (1985). Clinical nurse specialist role evaluation. *Oncology Nursing Forum, 12*(2), 62–66.

Henke, C. (1980). Emerging roles of the nurse in oncology. *Seminars in Oncology, 7*(1), 4–8.

Hennessey, S., & Wright, C. (1980). Oncology nurse education: The first step. *The Journal of Continuing Education in Nursing, 11*(1), 24–28.

Hilkemeyer, R. (1982). A historical perspective in cancer nursing. *Oncology Nursing Forum, 9*(2), 47–56.

Horvitz, I., & Trigg, J. (1986). Registered nurses and nursing students learn together in a cancer nursing course. *Nurse Educator, 11*(5), 37.

Howell, S. (1986). Continuing education in oncology nursing. *Journal of Continuing Education in Nursing, 17*, 119–121.

Itano, J., & Miller, C. (1990). Learning needs of Oncology Nursing Society members. *Oncology Nursing Forum, 17*, 697–703.

Krohner, K., & Spitak, A. (1992). Cancer nursing education in the community hospital: Principles and practice. *Oncology Nursing Forum, 19*, 783–790.

Mauksch, I. (1989). Understanding our past to build our future. *Oncology Nursing Forum, 16*, 483–487.

McGee, R. (1988). Survey of graduate programs in cancer nursing. *Oncology Nursing Forum, 15*, 90–96.

McGee, R., Powell, M., Broadwell, D., & Clark, J. (1987). A delphi survey of oncology clinical nurse specialist competencies. *Oncology Nursing Forum, 14*(2), 29–34.

McMillan, S. (1987). Program evaluation. *Oncology Nursing Forum, 14*(5), 67–70.

McMillan, S. (1988). Survey of graduate education programs in cancer nursing. *Oncology Nursing Forum, 15,* 825–831.

Mooney, M., & Dudas, S. (1987). Undergraduate independent study in cancer nursing. *Oncology Nursing Forum, 14*(1), 51–53.

Moore, I., Piper, B., Dodd, M., & Hudes, M. (1987). Measuring oncology nursing practice: Results from one graduate program. *Oncology Nursing Forum, 14*(1), 45–49.

Nevidjon, B., & Deatrich, J. (1985). An oncology clinical elective. *Oncology Nursing Forum, 12*(5), 57–59.

Oishi, N., Oki, G., Itano, J., Stringfellow, L., & Kurren, O. (1986). Professional schools team students to improve oncology care. *Nursing and Health Care, 7,* 446–449.

Oncology Nursing Society. (1989). *Standards of oncology nursing education: Generalist and advanced practice levels.* Pittsburgh, PA: Author.

Paulen, A. (1985). Practice issues for the oncology clinical nurse specialist. *Oncology Nursing Forum, 12*(2), 37–39.

Peterson, R. (1956). Federal grants for education in cancer nursing. *Nursing Outlook, 4,* 103–105.

Piemme, J. (1985). Oncology nurse clinical specialist education. *Oncology Nursing Forum, 12*(2), 45–48.

Piper, B. (1981). Continuing education programs in cancer nursing annual update and survey results. *Oncology Nursing Forum, 8*(3), 68–72.

Quinn-Casper, P., & Holmgren, C. (1987). Enhancing cancer nursing concepts in undergraduate curricula. *Cancer Nursing, 10,* 274–278.

Reed-Ash, C. (1988). Cancer nursing then and now. *Cancer Nursing, 11,* 1.

Siehl, S. (1982). The clinical nurse specialist in oncology. *Nursing Clinics of North America, 17,* 753–761.

Spross, J. (1983). An overview of the oncology clinical nurse specialist role. *Oncology Nursing Forum, 10*(3), 54–58.

Spross, J., & Donoghue, M. (1984). The future of the oncology clinical nurse specialist. *Oncology Nursing Forum, 11*(1), 74–78.

Welch-McCaffrey, D. (1986). Role performance issues for oncology clinical nurse specialists. *Cancer Nursing, 9,* 287–294.

Yasko, J. (1983). A survey of oncology clinical nursing specialists. *Oncology Nursing Forum, 10*(1), 25–30.

PART IV

Research on the Profession of Nursing

Chapter 9

Moral Competency

VIRGINIA R. CASSIDY
SCHOOL OF NURSING
NORTHERN ILLINOIS UNIVERSITY

CONTENTS

This is the third review in the area of nursing ethics that has appeared in the *Annual Review of Nursing Research*. Gortner's (1985) review of the work on ethical inquiry covered the literature until 1982 and was focused on the philosophical foundations of three issues: the professional roles of healer and scientist, the protection of human subjects, and peer and institutional review of research. In contrast to Gortner, Ketefian (1989) reviewed the empirical research on moral reasoning and ethical practice in nursing, covering the period from 1983 to early 1987. The themes of Ketefian's review were the processes employed by nurses in making moral choices and the decisions that nurses make in situations involving ethical dilemmas.

For this review, 38 empirical studies of nursing students and practicing nurses, published in the professional literature between 1987 and mid-1994, were selected for inclusion; studies were limited to those involving the use of human subjects. Themes similar to those of Ketefian (1989) appear in this review; however, studies in which nursing students and practicing nurses responded to the actual ethical circumstances in their education and/or practice are included. This inclusion adds a new dimension to understanding the breadth of ethical situations inherent in the profession and can provide direction to both nursing educators and practitioners for examining the ethical state of nursing. Dissertation research of nursing studies was reviewed because it adds a richness to the analysis and provides some perspective for anticipating future trends in nursing ethics research. In addition to the 38 studies from journals, 31 dissertations were included in the review. Data bases searched included Cumulative Index to Nursing and Allied Health Literature (CINAHL), Educational Resources Information Center (ERIC), and MEDLINE.

ORGANIZING FRAMEWORK

The perspective for this review is provided by the construct of moral competency. Moral competency, as described by Rest (1982), has four integrated critical elements that underlie moral action: sensitivity to the moral components of a situation, the formation of judgments about the situational components, the formulation of an intention to act in the situation, and the behavior necessary to execute the morally required action that the situation requires. Rest stated that moral development requires proficiency in all four of the critical elements that comprise moral competency. He suggested that the utility of a moral competency model lies in synthesizing the processes needed to understand moral development as "an ensemble of processes, rather than a single, unitary process" (Rest, 1982, p. 29).

As it is used in the context of this review, moral competency involves not only the ability to recognize the moral aspects of situations but also the cognitive and affective processes necessary for making decisions about those situations. Because much of the study of nursing ethics has involved the use of case studies or scenarios that incorporate ethical dilemmas, it is important to consider actions that nurses purport that they would take in those situations and the situational factors that may influence actions in positive or negative ways. Moral behavior is used in the broadest sense so that investigators who addressed the ethical aspects of education as well as practice are included.

Moral competency has been suggested as an important aspect in socializing nurses for their obligations in professional practice (Baker, 1987) and in delineating the responsibilities of nursing leaders (Cassidy & Koroll, 1994). This framework also can be useful in evaluating the current status of the research on nursing ethics and in providing direction for future inquiries. In the discussion of specific investigations that follows, for example, it will become evident that little work has yet to be done on the elements of moral intention and moral behavior. In some studies the element of moral sensitivity is addressed; however, in the majority of studies the focus is on the formation of moral judgments.

The review of the studies is divided into two broad sections, based on the subjects who were studied: nursing students and practicing nurses. In addition, studies are grouped to reflect a conceptualization of the moral competency model in order to demonstrate which of its elements have been emphasized in the studies reviewed. Not all findings from the studies can be presented, and the placement of studies in a particular section is based on its fit with the moral competency model and other similar works. That studies could be placed in more than one section is acknowledged.

CONCEPTUAL AND METHODOLOGICAL ISSUES

Broad concepts related to theoretical orientation, measurement of variables, and designs of ethics research in nursing are explored below in order to present a context for understanding the knowledge gained and the issues raised from the extant research.

Conceptual Orientation

Historically, the research on ethics in nursing has been considered primarily from a cognitive developmental approach. This approach was influenced almost exclusively by the work of Kohlberg (1976) until about 1990. Kohlberg proposed a moral development model based on a justice perspective in which stages of moral development are presented as sequential and invariate (Parker, 1990) and represent moral development changes from a preconventional to a conventional to a principled approach for addressing moral problems. Studies of nursing ethics have relied heavily on Kohlberg's justice framework, employed paper-and-pencil instruments that were developed from his justice perspective, and were implemented using quantitative methodologies (Cassidy, 1991).

More recently, the cognitive developmental paradigm employed in nursing ethics research has shifted from Kohlberg's ethic of justice to Gilligan (1977, 1982), who posited an ethic of care. On the basis of her studies of women, Gilligan also described moral development in stages but focused on the interpersonal elements that influenced women's evolution as moral agents. According to Gilligan, moral development begins with the stage of "orientation to individual survival," moves to the stage of "goodness as self-sacrifice," and finally, takes to a "morality as nonviolence" perspective.These stages parallel the preconventional, conventional, and principled stages of Kohlberg's model. The use of Gilligan's paradigm as a framework for research requires designs and data collection methods that lend themselves to more interactive, qualitative investigational techniques; these techniques have been reflected in some of the most recent nursing studies.

Measurement of Variables

Ketefian (1989) reported that three instruments, Rest's (1975) Defining Issues Test (DIT), Crisham's (1981) Nursing Dilemma Test (NDT), and Ketefian's (1981) Judgments about Nursing Decisions (JAND), were the most frequently used instruments in the studies included in her review. For the nursing studies reported in this review using paper-and-pencil instruments, this observation is still accurate. Ketefian (1989) provided a detailed description of these instruments; some additional psychometric information about them and their use is presented below.

Duckett et al. (1992) have raised numerous questions about how the DIT scores in nursing studies have been used and interpreted. Although reaffirming the reliability and validity of the DIT in more than 1,000 studies, they have challenged the conclusion of several authors that the instrument is not appropriate for use with nurses or nursing students. Among the issues they raised were the following: inappropriate comparisons of raw scores with percentile scores, both within analyses and in reference to normative data; comparisons of data from nursing students with an inappropriate normative group; misinterpretation of scores that fell within the "conventional" level as representative of "principled" thinking; the unfounded assertion that nurses score lower on the DIT than other groups; and, the overgeneralization of findings from small samples.

Corley and Selig (1992) reported that the internal consistency reliability for the principled thinking score of NDT in their study of critical care nurses was .36, in comparison to the .57 reported by Crisham (1981). In addition, they raised some issues about the validity of the NDT vignettes developed in 1979 in light of the numerous changes that have occurred in health care since that time. They also suggested that attempts to improve the usefulness of the NDT as a research instrument be undertaken by the addition of information and/or the addition of new vignettes.

Oddi and Cassidy (1994) raised several issues related to the use of the JAND in their investigations of nursing students and master's-prepared nurses. Among these issues were the inability to discriminate levels of moral reasoning among the groups studied, low or minimally acceptable levels of reliability in the original scales of the JAND, and the persistence of low reliability coefficients in the idealistic scale after the elimination of unreliable items. Questions also were raised about the validity of predetermining responses to questions of what a nurse would actually do when confronted with an ethical dilemma and the representativeness of the situations included in the instrument.

Research Designs

Studies included in this review reflect some shift from a quantitative approach to a qualitative approach. In the 1989 review, Ketefian cited only one qualitative study, whereas 26 are included here. Of note is that in all of the studies of nursing students ($N = 29$) except one (Candy, 1991), researchers continued to employ quantitative designs that were either descriptive, exploratory, or quasi-experimental. Studies of practicing nurses ($N = 40$) represented more of a quantitative-qualitative mix, with 18 reporting the use of descriptive or exploratory designs, 20 reporting qualitative aspects, and 2 reporting aspects of quantitative and qualitative approaches.

Sample sizes showed great variance, and few investigators reported the use of random sampling. In the studies of nursing students, sample sizes ranged from 51 to 2,209; randomly selected samples were reported in four cases (Cassidy & Oddi, 1988, 1991; Eddy, Elfrink, Weis, & Schank, 1994; Jordon, 1991). The studies were almost exclusively about baccalaureate nursing students ($n = 27$); Schuldenfrei (1990) studied only associate-degree students. Five other studies included associate-degree students as subjects (Cassells & Redman, 1989; Cassidy & Oddi, 1988, 1991; Daniel, Adams, & Smith, 1994; Oddi & Cassidy, 1994), and five included graduate students (Cassidy & Oddi, 1988, 1991; Hoover, 1991; Oddi & Cassidy, 1994; Wiley, Heath, & Acklin, 1988). Comparison groups in these studies included faculty or educational administrators (Hilbert, 1987; Kennedy, 1989; Stone, 1989), nonnursing undergraduate students (Mustapha & Seybert, 1989), counseling students (Hoover, 1991), medical students (Peter & Gallop, 1994), graduates of a baccalaureate program

(Schank & Weis, 1989), and master's-prepared nurses (Cassidy & Oddi, 1988, 1991; Oddi & Cassidy, 1994).

The subjects in the studies of nursing students were primarily women; men were reported as subjects in only eight studies (Daniel et al., 1994; Eddy, Eifrink, Weis, & Schank, 1994; Frisch, 1987; Hilbert, 1987; Mustapha & Seybert, 1989; Schank & Weis, 1989; Thurston, Flood, Shupe, & Gerald, 1989; Wehrwein, 1990) and represented between 7% and 18% of the groups investigated. The cultural/ethnic characteristics of students were reported only by Daniel et al. (1994), Eddy et al. (1994), and Hilbert (1987); African Americans, Asians, Hispanics, and Native Americans represented between 0.8% and 32.1% of these samples.

In the studies of practicing nurses, sample sizes ranged from 8 to 687. Randomly selected samples were reported in seven quantitative (Bell, 1991; Berger, Severson, & Chvatal, 1991; Cady, 1991; Miller, Beck, & Adams, 1991; Miya, 1990; Raines, 1992; Stoll, 1989) and two qualitative (O'Connor, 1991; Shipps, 1988) studies. All studies included registered nurses as all or a portion of the sample studied, and the majority of subjects were staff nurses. Samples represented nurses primarily from acute care settings; the practice areas represented most frequently included critical care (Chase, 1990; Cooper, 1991; Corley & Selig, 1992; Erlen & Frost, 1991; Holly, 1993; Soderberg & Norberg, 1993; Zalumas, 1989), medical-surgical (Davis, 1989, 1991; Erlen & Frost, 1991; Ferrell, Eberts, McCaffery, & Grant, 1991; Holly, 1993; Uden, Norberg, Lindseth, & Marhaug, 1992), neonatal intensive care (Chally, 1990; Raines, 1992), and oncology (Astrom, Jansson, Norberg, & Hallberg, 1993; Carney, 1987; Ferrell et al., 1991; O'Connor, 1991; Uden et al., 1992). Several studies were focused on or included nurses in home health care, public health, community health and/or hospice (Andrews, 1988; DeLa-Cruz, 1991; Duncan, 1992; Ferrell et al., 1991; Hatfield, 1991; Taylor, Ferrell, Grant, & Cheyney, 1993). Comparison groups included in several studies were composed of pharmacists and dentists (Miya, 1990), patients (Taylor et al., 1993), physicians (Burgess, Jacobson, Thompson, Baker, & Grant, 1990; Grundstein-Amado, 1992; Soderberg & Norberg, 1993), and social workers, counselors, and law enforcement and corrections officers (Burgess et al., 1990).

The inclusion of men who were practicing nurses was reported in 12 studies; men represented less than 25% of the sample in all studies in which they were included (Berger et al., 1991; Cady, 1991; Carney, 1987; Chase, 1990; Erlen & Frost, 1991; Ferrell et al., 1991; Garritson, 1988; Millette, 1993; Soderberg & Norberg, 1993; Wilson, 1991). The cultural/ethnic diversity of subjects was seldom reported. In five studies reporting cultural or ethnic data, only four included subjects other than Caucasians (Burgess et al., 1990; Garritson, 1988; Taylor et al., 1993); percentages for subgroups were not reported.

NURSING EDUCATION AND NURSING STUDENTS

Investigations of students can be divided into six subsections that reflect the elements of moral competency. Moral sensitivity is reflected in the subsections on ethics in the curriculum and the values of faculty and students; the formation of moral judgments is reflected in the subsections on instructional interventions and overall moral reasoning. Intent to act is addressed in the subsection on situational experiences, and moral action is addressed in the subsection on academic behavior.

Ethics in the Curriculum

Investigations that reflect an assessment of how moral sensitivity is developed in nursing students through curricular design were conducted by Cassells and Redman (1989), Haywood (1989), Kennedy (1989), and Stone (1989). In a national survey of students ($n = 1467$) and graduates ($n = 742$) of baccalaureate, associate degree, and diploma programs, Cassells and Redman (1989) provide a broad perspective on how ethics may or may not be recognized in undergraduate nursing curricula. Although 66% of the students and graduates of the programs reported completing coursework in ethics and 38% of them stated that it was required in the curriculum, 85% of the deans of these programs reported that ethics content was required and 75% of them reported that ethics content was integrated into nursing courses. The discrepancy in these findings may have resulted from different conceptions of what comprises ethics instruction and the inability of subjects to recall specific details of ethics content accurately.

In Stone's (1989) descriptive study of master's ($n = 143$) and doctorate ($n = 45$) nursing programs, faculty respondents gave opinions about nursing ethics and described the extent to which ethics content was taught in their programs. In telephone interviews, the majority of the faculty (72%) reported that ethics content was integrated into the curricula. In addition, Stone noted that few (1%) of the faculty were prepared to teach ethics content; this conclusion also was supported by findings from Cassells and Redman (1989) and Kennedy (1989). These self-reports provide an overview of how ethics instruction is approached in graduate curricula but do not provide a basis for determining the emphasis placed on ethics content in specific courses.

Haywood (1989) and Kennedy (1989) reported conflicting findings in their investigations of the effects of ethics content integrated into baccalaureate curricula versus discrete ethics courses. Kennedy found no differences in the level of moral reasoning on DIT scores nor knowledge of ethics on JAND scores among four groups of senior baccalaureate nursing students ($n = 80$). Haywood reported that senior nursing students who completed a discrete course in ethics scored higher at the postconventional level of moral reasoning [Defining Issues Test—Principled Reasoning scores (DIT-P scores)] than did students who had ethics integrated into the curriculum. The size of the sample in Haywood's study was not reported. Information on the comparability of the groups studied in both of these investigations was not reported and may account for the discrepancy in these findings.

Moral Sensitivity in Faculty and Nursing Students

The differences in moral sensitivity, defined as professional values, between baccalaureate nursing students and nursing faculty were studied by Eddy et al. (1994) and Thurston et al. (1989); Schank and Weis (1989) examined the relationship of the professional values of baccalaureate students and graduate nurses compared to the values reflected in the *Code for Nurses* (American Nurses Association, 1985). Weis et al. (Weis, Schank, Eddy, & Elfrink,1993) reported an analysis of the congruence between program objectives and the essential values identified by the American Association of Colleges of Nursing (AACN).

Schank and Weis (1989) reported no significant differences in values statements between students ($n = 138$) and graduates ($n = 61$) of secular and nonsecular baccalaureate programs but concluded that the subjects had not fully developed a professional value orientation. Eddy et al. (1994) reported significant differences in values statements between faculty and students in baccalaureate nursing programs, but no differences between the faculty ($n = 317$) and the students ($n = 636$) in public versus private institutions were noted. Thurston et al. (1989) reported significant differences in values statements between faculty ($n = 53$) and students ($n = 320$) in a baccalaureate nursing program; they reported that faculty and students chose the same AACN essential values as their most important ones but ranked them differently. Weis et al. (1993) concluded that, based on the reports of deans from 10 public and 16 private associate, baccalaureate, and graduate programs, the majority of programs participating in their study had objectives that reflected a least one of the AACN essential values.

The strengths of the Eddy et al. (1994) and the Weis et al. (1993) studies lie in the continuation of a program of research on professional values initiated by Schank and Weis in 1989, the use of cross-sectional random sampling, and the use of multivariate approaches in data collection. The findings are limited, however, to baccalaureate programs and subjects who are predominantly Caucasian women. Thurston et al. (1989) noted, as limitations of their study, the inclusion of a convenience sample of women faculty and students in one baccalaureate program and the lack of established reliability and validity on the AACN essential values.

Effects of Instructional Interventions

A cognitive developmental perspective was evident in studies on the effects of specific instruction in the formulation of moral judgments about ethical situations in baccalaureate nursing students. The results of five quasi-experimental studies were consistent in the lack of significant difference between experimental and control groups on the DIT (Frisch, 1987; Guice, 1992; Hembree, 1988), the JAND (Turner, 1990), and the Controversial Issues in Health Care Survey (Pederson, 1992) scores. Sample sizes in these studies ranged from 51 to 145; all samples were selected using nonprobability approaches. Treatment variables were unique to each study and included value analysis (Frisch, 1987), concept analysis (Guice, 1992), discussions of moral dilemmas (Hembree, 1988), structured controversy techniques (Pederson, 1992), and guided design instruction (Turner, 1990). The exposure to treatment variables varied across studies from several hours (Turner, 1990) to a 5-week course (Hembree, 1988) to a course taught over an academic term (Frisch, 1987; Pederson, 1992; Turner, 1990).

Rest (1982) has suggested that a single course in ethics may have little effect on moral judgments and that college students, in general, have a difficult time discerning principled thinking. These observations may account for the consistent lack of significant findings in this group of studies; in addition, some of the interventions employed in these studies provided a very brief exposure to ethics content (Hembree, 1988; Turner, 1990). Rest also discussed the importance of determining the students' stage of moral development in designing ethics content so that this content can be appreciated and assimilated by the students; in these studies it is not possible to determine if the moral development stage of the subjects was a consideration in designing the treatment variables.

Assessment of Ability to Make Moral Judgments

Comparisons in the ability of students to make moral judgments were made in eight exploratory studies between nurses and nonnurses (Hoover, 1991; Mustapha & Seybert, 1989), entering and graduating associate-degree students (Schuldenfrei, 1990), basic and RN degree–completion students (Wehrwein, 1990), basic and transfer students (Moore, 1991), associate-degree, generic baccalaureate, RN degree–completion, and master's degree students (Cassidy & Oddi, 1988, 1991) and associate-degree, generic baccalaureate, RN degree–completion, master's degree students, and master's-prepared nurses (Oddi & Cassidy, 1994). Sample sizes in these studies ranged from 130 to 266; sample sizes were not reported by Hoover or Schuldenfrei. In six of the eight studies no significant differences were found between groups on DIT (Schuldenfrei,

1990; Wehrwein, 1990), JAND (Cassidy & Oddi, 1988, 1991; Moore, 1991; Wehrwein, 1990), and Ethical Judgment Scale (EJS) (Hoover, 1991) scores. Mustapha and Seybert (1989) reported that women had significantly higher DIT-P scores than men did. They also found that liberal arts students in an integrated curriculum had significantly higher DIT-P scores than nursing students did. Oddi and Cassidy (1994) reported differences only between RN degree–completion students and master's-prepared nurses on the realistic scale of the JAND.

As no experimental manipulation was employed in these investigations, the lack of differences between the groups studied may have arisen from a variety of threats to internal and external validity. Although sample sizes appeared to be adequate in this group of studies, overall, the groups studied may have, in fact, been comparable in their ability to make moral judgments. Another possible explanation may be a lack of sensitivity (Hoover, 1991) or inadequate reliability and validity (Cassidy & Oddi, 1988, 1991; Oddi & Cassidy, 1994) in the measures of moral judgments.

Only Peter and Gallop (1994) investigated the construct of caring, as it is defined by Gilligan (1977), among nursing ($n = 68$) and medical ($n = 51$) students. They concluded that their findings supported Gilligan's model because the women subjects used care considerations more often than the men did. They also reported that an eclectic approach to moral reasoning was the representative model in these nursing and medical students because care and justice perspectives were seen in both groups; these findings are supported in studies of practicing nurses (Chally, 1990; Chase, 1990; Millette, 1993).

Situational Experiences

In three investigations, students' moral intentions in specific rather than general situations were considered; the situations involved caring for persons with AIDS (PWA) (Jordon, 1991; Wiley et al., 1988) and individuals with a do-not-resuscitate (DNR) order (Candy, 1991). Jordon (1991) reported that baccalaureate students ($n = 311$) were reluctant or unwilling to care for PWA due to fear of exposure to AIDS, and Wiley et al. (1988) reported the same findings in master's-degree ($n = 47$), RN degree–completion ($n = 18$), and generic baccalaureate ($n = 77$) students. Jordan (1991) further reported that students overwhelmingly indicated that they would care for PWA and that PWA were entitled to the same care as any other patients. In contrast, Wiley et al. (1988) reported that 21% to 45% of the student groups studied communicated that they would "probably" or "definitely" refuse to care for patients who were seropositive for human immunodeficiency virus (HIV). Candy (1991) reported that students ($N = 71$) in England perceived nurses to have little influence in decisions related to DNR status but that DNR status did not equate with the withdrawal of nursing care. These few studies of moral intent raise questions about behaviors that subjects might exhibit in actual situations. Rest (1982) has suggested that what individuals propose they ought do for moral reasons is not necessarily what they do in reality.

Unethical Academic Behavior

An area of relatively little investigation in the domain of moral judgments and behavior among nursing students is that of unethical academic behavior. Unethical academic behavior involves various forms of cheating in classroom and clinical coursework on the part of students (Daniel et al., 1994; Hilbert, 1987; Sheer, 1989) and how students perceive inappropriate actions or communications among faculty (Theis, 1988). Grade point average (GPA), personality traits, and demographic characteristics were used as predictors of unethical classroom and clinical behaviors. In analyses of self-reported unethical behaviors among baccalaureate students ($N = 210$), Hilbert (1987) found no relationship between predictor variables and scores of unethical behaviors on the Hilbert Unethical Behavior Scale (HUBS) but did report differences in unethical clinical behaviors by ethnic background and a significant positive relationship between unethical classroom and clinical behaviors. Sheer's (1989) findings were similar to Hilbert's in that personality variables were not significant predictors of overall unethical behaviors among baccalaureate students ($n = 308$) but were predictive of unethical clinical behaviors. Daniel et al. (1994) supported the hypothesis that associate-degree and baccalaureate students' ($N = 190$) perceptions of and attitudes toward their peers were significantly correlated with perceptions of their peers' participation in academic misconduct. In the study of senior baccalaureate students' ($N = 204$) perceptions of faculty, Theis (1988) related that the majority of subjects reported between one and four examples of what they perceived as unethical conduct on the part of faculty. These examples represented a perceived lack of faculty respect for students in classroom and clinical situations and for patients in the clinical setting.

Hilbert (1987) and Sheer (1989) employed the HUBS in their study and were able to differentiate among subgroups on one scale, which suggests validity in predicting unethical clinical behaviors; further development of this instrument would provide a valuable tool for other investigations of unethical academic behavior. The Daniel et al. (1994) multivariate analysis and exploration of motivation in the investigation of unethical behavior suggests additional factors for consideration in future research, as the use of individual personality characteristics seem to have little predictive value (Hilbert, 1987; Sheer, 1989). The Theis (1988) study of how students perceive faculty behaviors opens a new area for ethics investigation and has implications for understanding how the behaviors "modeled" by faculty may influence students' own behavior. Theis suggests further work in students' perceptions of ethical behaviors in faculty and instrument development in this area.

NURSING PRACTICE AND PRACTICING NURSES

The research related to nurses and their practice can be divided into four sections: the moral sensitivity of nurses, assessment of nurses' ability to make moral judgments, the ethic of care versus the ethic of justice in moral reasoning, and situational experiences.

Moral Sensitivity in Nurses

Andrews (1988), Bell (1991), Berger et al. (1991), Davis (1991), Garritson (1988), Miller et al. (1991), Miya (1990), Raines (1992), Smith (1989), and Supples (1993) conducted studies related to moral sensitivity in practicing nurses. Employing ethnographic interviews, Supples described the situations of professional incompetence or substandard practice that staff nurses and nursing administrators ($N = 38$) considered cause for concern. She found that, despite the severity of some of the situations, mild, if any, disciplinary action was reported by subjects. The proportion of staff nurses and nursing administrators in this study was not reported, and subjects communicated personal knowledge of these issues. It is not possible to determine the extent to which staff nurses had access to all relevant information regarding disciplinary action.

Bell (1991) investigated the manner in which nurses ($N = 129$) defined the advocacy role and concluded that nurses recognized the need to defend patients' rights but they may frequently be unable to enact the role. Support for this finding may be found in the Andrew (1988), Davis (1991), and Smith (1989) judgments that current nursing education prepared nurses to cope with ethical dilemmas to only a slight or moderate degree and has little influence on nurses' own professional values and code of ethics. In addition, Berger et al. (1991) stated that the subjects ($N = 156$) in their study reported encountering few ethical issues in their practice. They deduced that this finding might be accounted for by low sensitivity to these issues. In a related finding from a state survey of practicing nurses ($N = 514$), Miller et al. (1991) reported that 60% of the sample were not familiar with the tenets of the *Code for Nurses* (American Nurses Association, 1985).

In response to hypothetical vignettes, Raines (1992) concluded that nurses ($N = 331$) had a hierarchy of values in which "doing right" and beneficence were ranked as the highest values among neonatal nurses, but there was a lack of congruence between the values chosen and the self-reports of behaviors that were implemented in practice. Garritson (1988) also reported that beneficence was the basis of responses to case vignettes in her study of psychiatric nurses ($N = 165$), and Miya (1990) reported that autonomy was the highest value held by nurses ($N = 180$), dentists ($N = 60$), and pharmacists ($N = 60$). Garritson further reported that responses were not consistent within subjects nor across situations and speculated that this finding may be accounted for by situational factors. Davis (1991) concluded that situational factors and the complexity and uncertainty of clinical circumstances influenced nurses' ($N = 27$) sensitivity to the ethics of their clinical practice; she also postulated that nurses may become desensitized to ethical dilemmas as a coping mechanism for their frustration in repeatedly confronting these dilemmas.

Researcher-developed instruments were employed in studies by Andrews (1988), Bell (1991), Berger et al. (1991), Garritson (1988), Miller et al. (1991), Miya (1990), and Raines (1992). In general, little or no data on the psychometric properties of these instruments were reported; procedures to establish content validity using expert panels were mentioned. Given the early stages of the development of these instruments and their limited use in data collection, the findings of these exploratory studies should be viewed as tentative. Further evaluation and development of these instruments is needed to establish their usefulness in future investigations.

Assessment of Nurses' Ability to Make Moral Judgments

Investigations of nurses' ability to form moral judgments about hypothetical situations were reported by Corley and Selig (1992), Hatfield (1991), Mahoney (1991), and Stoll (1989). The DIT was used by Mahoney and Stoll; the NDT was used by Corley and Selig and Hatfield. Conflicting findings about the effects of demographic and personality characteristics on moral judgments were reported in these studies. Mahoney (1991) and Corley and Selig (1992) reported no correlation between education and scores on the DIT and NDT for nurses working in acute care ($N = 81$) and critical care ($N = 75$), respectively. Stoll (1989) found that educational level and perceptions of organizational climate were predictors of DIT scores among nurses in a Veterans Administration hospital ($N = 345$). Corley and Selig (1992) and Hatfield (1991) reported significant correlations between years of experience and NDT scores in critical care nurses and home health care nurses; no such relationship was found by Hatfield for public health or hospice nurses. Inconsistent findings in these studies may be attributed to low internal consistency reliability in the NDT and the relevance of the content of its items to current practice, as discussed earlier.

Differences in age, experience with ethical dilemmas, and education may also contribute to lack of consistent findings. For example, Rest (1982) related that formal academic education is the most consistent correlate to moral judgment; however, the specific experiences and conditions that promote this develop-ment are not known.

Three interrelated themes were identified in the 12 qualitative studies of nurses' ability to form moral judgments: decision-making processes (Dela-Cruz, 1991; Dewolf, 1989; Grundstein-Amado, 1992), the context of decisions (Arndt, 1994; Astrom et al., 1993; Beaugard, 1990; Dela-Cruz, 1991; Holly, 1993; Viens, 1992), and conflicts in relationships (Beaugard, 1990; Case, 1991; Duncan, 1992; Grundstein-Amado, 1992; Holly, 1993; Soderberg & Norberg, 1993; Uden et al., 1992; Wellard, 1992; Zalumas, 1989). Decision-making processes were represented as logically interconnected cognitive processes that began with problem identification and progressed to efforts to evaluate the course of action chosen. Two models of decision making were developed in grounded-theory investigations of home-care nurses (N = 21) (Dela-Cruz, 1991) and nurses in acute medical settings (N not reported) (Dewolf, 1989). The Grundstein-Amado (1992) findings supported a five-stage decision-making model used by nurses (n = 9) and physicians (n = 9). The findings of these studies appear to be limited to the groups studied, but the Dela-Cruz (1991) study of home-care nurses is important in identifying the ethical issues in the home-care management of patients and in clarifying how decisions are made about the management of these issues.

Contextual factors that positively or negatively affect the ethical aspects of care were reported in studies of home-care nurses (Dela-Cruz, 1991), nurses employed in acute care settings (Arndt, 1994; Beaugard, 1990; Holly, 1993; Shipps, 1988) and clinics (Astrom et al., 1993), and nurse practitioners (Viens, 1992). Among the contextual factors cited as important were institutional con-straints or the practice environment (Arndt, 1994; Dela-Cruz, 1991; Holly, 1993; Viens, 1992), the nurse-patient relationship (Arndt, 1994; Astrom et al., 1993; Beaugard, 1990; Dela-Cruz, 1991), the health status of the patient, and legal and economic factors (Dela-Cruz, 1991). In these qualitative studies, some insight into the actual experiences of nurses in addressing the ethical issues in selected aspects of care can be gained. In addition to these studies, the context of ethical situations is also identified as an important aspect in several other studies (Davis, 1991; Grundstein-Amado, 1992; Holly, 1993).

Conflicts in relationships and nurses' experiences with moral conflicts were evident in the analyses of several studies. Conflicts with physicians or with physicians' decisions (Davis, 1989; Holly, 1993; Soderberg & Norberg, 1993; Uden et al., 1992; Wellard, 1992; Zalumas, 1989) were the areas repre-sented most frequently. Conflicts also arose from interactions with other nurses

(Wellard, 1992), with patients (Duncan, 1992; Wellard, 1992), and with administrators (Wellard, 1992; Zalumas, 1989). Conflict in perceptions of nurses' roles was reported by Beaugard (1990) and Carney (1987). The source of these conflicts, particularly those between physicians and nurses, was identified as a difference in professional and gender perspectives. Davis (1989) and Holly (1993) also reported that nurses were most concerned with patients' rights in their descriptions of conflicts.

Nurses' experiences with and reactions to these conflicts were described by Case (1991), Holly (1993), and Erlen and Frost (1991). Case (1991) portrayed these experiences with conflicts as having six essential features: choice, advocacy, autonomy, pain and suffering, values, and relationships. In the Holly (1993) study, nurses viewed patients as being exploited or excluded from decision making, and this produced anguish in the nurses. Powerlessness was reported as the shared experience among subjects by Erlen and Frost (1991); these situations produced anger, frustration, and exhaustion. These findings were also supported by Raines (1992).

In these self-reports of lived experience with ethical dilemmas, nurses consistently identified communications and interpersonal relationships in institutional hierarchies as negative influences in addressing ethical matters. Both Holly (1993) and Erlen and Frost (1991), however, suggest that their findings could be attributed to the study of volunteers, who might recently have had particularly distressing experiences with ethical dilemmas.

An Ethic of Care versus an Ethic of Justice in Moral Reasoning

Six studies represent specific attempts to describe or compare approaches to moral reasoning based on Kohlberg's (1976) versus Gilligan's (1977) model of moral development; one compared a principle-oriented framework with an ethic of care (Cooper, 1991). Five researchers employed a qualitative approach to their investigations (Chally, 1990; Chase, 1990; Cooper, 1991; Millette, 1993; O'Connor, 1991), and two employed a quantitative approach (Cady, 1991; Wilson, 1991). The groups studied in these investigations were described as nurses working in specialty areas such as neonatal intensive care (*N* not reported) (Chally, 1990), oncology (O'Connor, 1991), and critical care (Chase, 1990; Cooper, 1991) or employed nurses from a geographic region (Cady, 1991; Millette, 1993; Wilson, 1991). Sample sizes ranged from 8 (Cooper, 1991) to 418 (Cady, 1991), but little detail was provided on other demographic characteristics. The findings of all studies were consistent in reporting an eclectic approach to moral reasoning in subjects.

All of these studies were reported in the past 5 years, which illustrates that the investigation of approaches to moral reasoning is a relatively new area of research interest in nursing ethics. Despite the fact that these studies were essentially done concurrently and employed different methodologies, the consistency in the findings suggests that nurses do not use one approach in their moral reasoning about clinical situations. These studies can serve as a basis for further refinement of methods to explore this aspect of ethical practice.

Situational Experiences

Three studies addressed issues related to the context and/or conflicts in nurses' moral judgments in specific situations, namely, cancer pain management (Ferrell et al., 1991; Taylor et al., 1993) and HIV testing in assailants and sexual assault victims (Burgess et al., 1990). In these studies, nurses experienced professional conflicts that were inter- and intrapersonal in trying to do what was best for patients to relieve pain without causing harm (Ferrell et al., 1991; Taylor et al., 1993) and in attempting to balance social good and personal rights in situations related to HIV status (Burgess et al., 1990).

The findings of Ferrell et al. (1991) and Taylor et al. (1993) are limited by the use of convenience sampling, relatively small sample sizes ($N = 53$; $N = 10$, respectively) and their descriptive methods. They do, however, corroborate the findings of other studies, that nurses may experience ethical conflict because of inadequate knowledge (Erlen & Frost, 1991; Raines, 1992). Although the sample of nurses in the study by Burgess et al. (1990) was large ($N = 230$), the findings are limited to emergency department nurses. In addition, questionnaires were mailed to individuals "likely to have contact with sexual assault victims and perpetrators" (Burgess et al., 1990, p. 331), but the number of nurses who had experience in providing direct care to HIV-positive individuals and PWA was not reported.

CONCLUSIONS AND RESEARCH DIRECTIONS

Although much can be learned from research using the framework of moral competency, much still needs to be learned, and much work is yet to be done in this field. As a body of scientific literature, the research in ethics lacks the rigor that one might expect in light of the number of nurses prepared to conduct scientific inquiries and the variety of methodological approaches now available and accepted as legitimate within the field. There is some indication that ethics research is becoming cumulative, but evidence of ongoing research programs among the investigators cited (i.e., Cassidy & Oddi, 1988, 1991; Oddi & Cassidy, 1994; Eddy et al., 1994; Schank & Weis, 1989; Thurston et al.,

1989) is minimal, and only one replication study (Cassidy & Oddi, 1991) was identified.

For studies using quantitative methods, few attempts to secure random samples were made. Students in baccalaureate programs and nurses practicing in hospitals are the primary groups studied, but assumptions about the homogeneity of these groups should be made with prudence. In addition, the characteristics of subjects were not always described sufficiently to understand the breadth of generalizations that can be made; rather, many investigators cautioned against generalizing findings beyond the group studied. The influence of gender and cultural and ethnic diversity has not received adequate systematic exploration in investigations of ethical matters as they relate to nursing students and practicing nurses.

In studies of students and practicing nurses, it appears that current educational processes are not sufficient to elevate the sensitivity of students to the level needed to address the diversity of ethical issues in practice. Inconsistency in the content, exposure, goals, and objectives of ethics instruction in nursing curricula, at both the undergraduate and graduate levels, is a matter that must be addressed by researchers, educators, and administrators in the profession.

Attempts to influence the moral judgments of students with isolated, short-term interventions, such as exposure to ethics content as a treatment variable, is shortsighted and reflects a somewhat simplistic view of a complex phenomenon. The cumulative lack of significant findings in quasi-experimental research suggests that more is to be learned about the factors that influence moral judgments, through descriptive and exploratory research, before meaningful interventions can be devised. If moral development involves processes, insights, and abilities that evolve over time, as Rest (1982) suggests, and if understanding this development is of importance to nurses, then attempts to investigate it as an ongoing, developmental process should be initiated.

Additional attention should he paid to the academic environment as an influence on moral judgments and moral behavior. The apparent willingness of some students to participate in academic misconduct raises concerns about the ethical standards that these nurses-to-be will embrace in their practice. Further, the need for nursing faculty to be role models for ethical decision making and behavior warrants thoughtful consideration in the academic community.

The preponderance of studies included here have been focused on the cognitive and affective facets of the moral competency model. Study of these aspects of moral competency continues to be important, and they should be used as the basis for understanding the actual behavior of students and nurses in ethical situations. Investigations of moral behavior should also incorporate the context in which this behavior occurs. Evidence of the effects of institutional hierarchies and interpersonal relationships on nurses' ability to behave in moral ways is accumulating; however, it does not appear that this evidence has been used as the basis for any change in organizational structure or role definition. It raises questions about whether or not ethical behavior is truly valued in the practice setting.

Issues in the measurement of ethical constructs remain problematic, and the issues have not been addressed adequately over time; both Gortner (1985) and Ketefian (1989) identified this as a concern. The construction of new instruments for measuring moral constructs, as reported by several investigators, can be viewed as positive steps. Further refinement and validation of these instruments, however, is needed to determine their utility in the measurement of ethical constructs (Cassidy, 1991)

The employment of qualitative approaches in the investigation of ethical matters has brought new perceptions of the real-life experiences, concerns, insights, and issues (Munhall, 1989) of practicing nurses. Allowing nurses to use their own voices in relating the ethics of their practice has provided a context for understanding the ethical milieu of the practice environment and acknowledging the humanity of the research endeavor (Ramos, 1989), and it is well suited to understanding the complexity and uncertainty inherent in ethical dilemmas. It is of concern, however, that this approach has not been employed in investigations of the moral competency of nursing students. Use of qualitative techniques in investigations of nursing students offers the potential for discerning the educational experiences that will better provide students with the knowledge, values, skills, and competencies for ethical practice.

The debate on the justice versus care perspectives of moral development continues. Gilligan's (1982) ethic of care has had wide appeal in nursing ethics research because it appears to address the issue of gender-specific morality raised by Kohlberg's study of males in the development of his ethic of justice model. Attempts to represent Gilligan's model as totally separate and distinct from Kohlberg's, however, may be overstated. In fact, the structure of both models is a three-stage configuration that is suggested as sequential; that is, one moves from level to level in an upwardly developmental mode. Direct comparisons of the structure of the two models highlight these similarities (Parker, 1990; Silva, 1990). In addition, in the substance of Gilligan's model she does not totally negate the applicability of the justice perspective to women nor totally confine the caring perspective to women; she suggests that at the highest level of moral reasoning there is a convergence of women's and men's development (Bloom, 1986).

The appeal of Gilligan's (1982) model in nursing is further highlighted by the conclusions drawn about some nursing studies in which few subjects were classified as principled thinkers within Kohlberg's framework. If one were to assume, however, that moral development is a human trait with variance similar to characteristics such as aptitudes and other personality characteristics (Anastasi, 1988), then the overall distribution of moral development scores would approximate a normal curve. The majority of individuals tested for this trait would have scores that cluster in the center of the distribution, representing a midrange or conventional level of moral development, with the number of cases at the low end (preconventional level) and the high end (principled level) of the distribution occurring less frequently. One might expect that nurses would be similar to other groups in the distribution of this characteristic. The issues, then, may lie more with the distribution of moral development stages in the nursing population than with the model used to describe this development.

Direct empirical comparisons of women's moral development using both Kohlberg's and Gilligan's (1977) models are few. The coexistence and the use of more than one perspective, be it justice, caring, or principle orientation, for addressing ethical issues is evident in the research reviewed here. On the basis of these findings, it appears that an eclectic approach is more likely to explain nurses' moral reasoning and behavior than an either/or (Kohlberg vs. Gilligan) approach. Consideration of other conceptualizations of caring, such as those posed by Noddings, Leininger, and Watson, may also be fruitful to explore in understanding this phenomenon in nursing ethics (Crowley, 1994; Eliason, 1993; Morse, Bottorff, Neander, & Solberg, 1991).

Issues raised in this review have been focused primarily on the methodological aspects of the studies selected for analysis. Addressing these issues in future investigations should be a priority for establishing a strong foundation for the investigation of nursing ethics. In addition, in her review on ethical inquiry, Gortner (1985) identified the need for investigations related to the ethical conduct of research, the surveillance of practice and research behaviors, and patients' and families' participation in making treatment decisions. The nature of this review precluded discussion of these topics, but they are important areas for nursing ethics research. A substantive body of literature exists in each of these areas; any of these topics could serve as the basis for integrative reviews and future nursing ethics research.

ACKNOWLEDGMENT

The assistance of Sue Lehman–Trzynka in the compilation of the bibliography for this chapter is gratefully acknowledged.

REFERENCES

American Nurses Association. (1985). *Code for nurses with interpretive statements.* Kansas City, MO: Author.

Anastasi, A. (1988). *Psychological testing* (6th ed.). New York: Macmillan.

Andrews, E. M. B. (1988). *Ethical dilemmas encountered by nurses employed by hospitals, community health agencies, and public schools* [CD-ROM]. Abstract from: SilverPlatter File: Dissertation Abstracts Item: 115616.

Arndt, M. (1994). Nurses' medication errors. *Journal of Advanced Nursing, 19,* 519–526.

Astrom, G., Jansson, L., Norberg, A., & Hallberg, I. R. (1993). Experienced nurses' narratives of their being in ethically difficult care situations. *Cancer Nursing, 16,* 179–187.

Baker, P. D. (1987). Moral competency: An essential element in the socialization of professional nurses. *Family and Community Health, 10*(1), 8–14.

Beaugard, C. R. (1990). *How hospital nurses reason about ethical dilemmas of practice* [CD-ROM]. Abstract from: SilverPlatter File: Dissertation Abstracts Item: 133626

Bell, L. (1991). Moral dilemmas in clinical practice. *Plastic Surgical Nursing, 11,* 176–180.

Berger, M. C., Severson, A., & Chvatal, R. (1991). Ethical issues in nursing. *Western Journal of Nursing Research, 13,* 514–521.

Bloom, A. H. (1986). Psychological ingredients of high-level moral thinking: A critique of the Kohlberg-Gilligan paradigm. *Journal for the Theory of Social Behaviour, 16,* 89–103.

Burgess, A. W., Jacobson, B., Thompson, J. E., Baker, T., & Grant, C. A. (1990). HIV testing of sexual assault populations: Ethical and legal issues. *Journal of Emergency Nursing, 16,* 331–338.

Cady, P. A. (1991). *An analysis of moral judgment in registered nurses: Principled reasoning versus caring values* [CD-ROM]. Abstract from: SilverPlatter File: Dissertation Abstracts Item: 152155

Candy, C. E. (1991). "Not for resuscitation": The student nurses' viewpoint. *Journal of Advanced Nursing, 16,* 138–146.

Carney, B. (1987). Bone marrow transplantation: Nurses' and physicians' perceptions of informed consent. *Cancer Nursing, 10,* 252–269.

Case, N. K. (1991). *A description of the meaning of moral conflict in pediatric nursing practice: Weaving the fabric of choice* [CD-ROM]. Abstract from: SilverPlatter File: Dissertation Abstracts Item: 152109

Cassells, J. M., & Redman, B. K. (1989). Preparing students to be moral agents in clinical nursing practice: Report of a national study. *Nursing Clinics of North America, 24,* 463–473.

Cassidy, V. R. (1991). Ethical responsibilities in nursing: Research findings and issues. *Journal of Professional Nursing, 7,* 112–118.

Cassidy, V. R., & Koroll, C. J. (1994). Ethical aspects of transformational leadership. *Holistic Nursing Practice, 41*(1), 41–47.

Cassidy, V. R., & Oddi, L. F. (1988). Professional autonomy and ethical decision making among graduate and undergraduate nursing majors. *Journal of Nursing Education, 27,* 405–410.

Cassidy, V. R., & Oddi, L. F. (1991). Professional autonomy and ethical decision making among graduate and undergraduate nursing majors: A replication. *Journal of Nursing Education, 30*, 149–151.

Chally, P. S. (1990). *Moral decision-making by neonatal intensive care nurses* [CD-ROM]. Abstract from: SilverPlatter File: Dissertation Abstracts Item: 142500

Chase, S. K. (1990). *Clinical judgment by critical care nurses: An ethnographic study* [CD-ROM]. Abstract from: SilverPlatter File: Dissertation Abstracts Item: 133606

Cooper, M. C. (1991). Principle-oriented ethics and the ethic of care: A creative tension. *Advances in Nursing Science, 14*(1), 22–31.

Corley, M. C., & Selig, P. M. (1992). Nurses moral reasoning: Using the nursing dilemma test. *Western Journal of Nursing Research, 4*, 380–388.

Crisham, P. (1981). Measuring moral judgment in nursing dilemmas. *Nursing Research, 30*, 104–110.

Crowley, M. A. (1994). The relevance of Noddings' ethics of care to the moral education of nurses. *Journal of Nursing Education, 33*, 74–80.

Daniel, L. G., Adams, B. N., & Smith, N. M. (1994). Academic misconduct among nursing students: A multivariate investigation. *Journal of Professional Nursing, 10*, 278–288.

Davis, A. J. (1989). Informed consent process in research protocols: Dilemmas for clinical nurses. *Western Journal of Nursing Research, 11*, 448–547.

Davis, A. J. (1991). The sources of a practice code of ethics for nurses. *Journal of Advanced Nursing, 16*, 1358–1362.

Dela-Cruz, F. A. (1991). *Managing patient care: A substantive theory of clinical decision making in home health care nursing* [CD-ROM]. Abstract from: SilverPlatter File: Dissertation Abstracts Item: 152062

Dewolf, M. S. (1989). *Clinical ethical decision-making: A grounded theory method* [CD-ROM]. Abstract from: SilverPlatter File: Dissertation Abstracts Item: 126481

Duckett, L., Rowan-Boyer, M, Ryden, M. B., Crisham, P., Savik, K., & Rest, J. T. (1992). Challenging misperceptions about nurses' moral reasoning. *Nursing Research, 41*, 324–331.

Duncan, S. M. (1992). Ethical challenge in community health nursing. *Journal of Advanced Nursing, 17*, 1035–1041.

Eddy, D. M., Elfrink, V., Weis, D., & Schank, M. J. (1994). Importance of professional nursing values: A national study of baccalaureate programs. *Journal of Nursing Education, 33*, 257–262.

Eliason, M. J. (1993). Ethics and transcultural nursing care. *Nursing Outlook, 41*, 225–228.

Erlen, J. A., & Frost, B. (1991). Nurses' perceptions of powerlessness in influencing ethical decisions. *Western Journal of Nursing Research, 13*, 397–407.

Ferrell, B. R., Eberts, M. T., McCaffery, M., & Grant, M. (1991). Clinical decision making and pain. *Cancer Nursing, 14*, 289– 297.

Frisch, N. C. (1987). Value analysis: A method for teaching nursing ethics and promoting the moral development of students. *Journal of Nursing Education, 26*, 328–332.

Garritson, S. H. (1988). Ethical decision making patterns. *Journal of Psychosocial Nursing, 26*(4), 22–29.

Gilligan, C. (1977). In a different voice: Women's conceptions of self and of morality. *Harvard Educational Review, 47*, 481–517.

Gilligan, C. (1982). *In a different voice: Psychological theory and women's development.* Cambridge, MA: Harvard University Press.

Gortner, S. R. (1985). Ethical inquiry. In H. H. Werley & J. J. Fitzpatrick (Eds.), *Annual Review of Nursing Research* (pp. 193–214). New York: Springer Publishing Co.

Grundstein-Amado, R. (1992). Differences in ethical decision-making processes among nurses and doctors. *Journal of Advanced Nursing, 17*, 129–137.

Guice, E. D. (1992). *The effect of instruction in concept analysis on critical thinking skills and moral reasoning decisions of senior baccalaureate nursing students* [CD-ROM]. Abstract from: SilverPlatter File: Dissertation Abstracts Item: 189978

Hatfield, P. G. (1991). *The relationship between levels of moral/ethical judgment, advocacy and autonomy among community health nurses* [CD-ROM]. Abstract from: SilverPlatter File: Dissertation Abstracts Item: 157043

Haywood, J. M. (1989). *The relationship of moral development stages to ethics content in nursing curricula* [CD-ROM]. Abstract from: SilverPlatter File: Dissertation Abstracts Item: 131260

Hembree, B. S. (1988). *The effect of moral dilemma discussions on moral reasoning levels of baccalaureate nursing students* [CDROM]. Abstract from: SilverPlatter File: Dissertation Abstracts Item: 115425

Hilbert, G. A. (1987). Academic fraud: Prevalence, practices and reasons. *Journal of Professional Nursing, 3*, 39–45.

Holly, C. M. (1993). The ethical quandaries of acute care nursing practice. *Journal of Professional Nursing, 9*, 110–115.

Hoover, R. M. (1991). *Relationship of sex-role identity and ethical orientation of graduate students in two helping professions: Counselors and nurses* [CD-ROM]. Abstract from: SilverPlatter File: Dissertation Abstracts Item: 159345

Jordon, J. C. (1991). *The relationship between baccalaureate nursing students' knowledge of AIDS, attitudes toward AIDS and willingness to care for people with AIDS* [CD-ROM]. Abstract from: SilverPlatter File: Dissertation Abstracts Item: 157042

Kennedy, P. H. (1989). *Curricular approaches to ethical instruction and the development of moral reasoning in baccalaureate nursing students* [CD-ROM]. Abstract from: SilverPlatter File: Dissertation Abstracts Item: 119019

Ketefian, S. (1981). Moral reasoning and moral behavior among selected groups of practicing nurses. *Nursing Research, 30*, 171–176.

Ketefian, S. (1989). Moral reasoning and ethical practice. In J. J. Fitzpatrick, R. L. Taunton, & J. Q. Benoliel (Eds.), *Annual Review of Nursing Research* (pp. 173–195). New York: Springer Publishing Co..

Kohlberg, L. (1976). Moral stages and moralization: The cognitive developmental approach. In T. Lickona (Ed.), *Moral development and behavior: Theory research and social issues* (pp. 32–53). New York: Holt, Rinehart, & Winston.

Mahoney, K. M. (1991). *Life experiences and moral judgment of registered nurses* [CD-ROM]. Abstract from: SilverPlatter File: Dissertation Abstracts Item: 156060

Miller, B. K., Beck, L., & Adams, D. (1991). Nurses' knowledge of the code for nurses. *Journal of Continuing Education in Nursing, 22*, 198–202.

Millette, B. E. (1993). Client advocacy and the moral orientation of nurses. *Western Journal of Nursing Research, 15*, 607–618.

Miya, P. A. (1990). *World views of health science faculty investigators: Biomedical ethical issues and principle in human subject research* [CD-ROM]. Abstract from: SilverPlatter File: Dissertation Abstracts Item: 135101

Moore, L. (1991). *A comparison of professional values in 2 different types of baccalaureate nursing students* [CD-ROM]. Abstract from: SilverPlatter File: Dissertation Abstracts Item: 157232

Morse, J. M., Bottorff, J., Neander, W., & Solberg, S. (1991). Comparative analysis of conceptualizations and theories of caring. *Image: The Journal of Nursing Scholarship, 23,* 119–126.

Munhall, P. L. (1989). Philosophical ponderings on qualitative research methods in nursing. *Nursing Science Ouarterly, 20,* 20–28.

Mustapha, S. A., & Seybert, J. A. (1989). Moral reasoning in college students: Implications for nursing education. *Journal of Nursing Education, 28,* 107–111.

O'Connor, K. E. (1991). *The ethical/moral language of cancer nurses* [CD-ROM]. Abstract from: ProQuest File: Dissertation Abstracts Item: 9123653

Oddi, L. F., & Cassidy, V. R. (1994). The JAND as a measure of nurses' perception of moral behaviors. *International Journal Nursing Studies, 31,* 37–47.

Parker, R. S. (1990). Measuring nurses' moral judgments. *Image: Journal of Nursing Scholarship, 22,* 213–218.

Pederson, C. (1992). Effects of structured controversy on students' perceptions of their skills in discussing controversial issues. *Journal of Nursing Education, 31,* 101–106.

Peter, E., & Gallop, R. (1994). The ethic of care: A comparison of nursing and medical students. *Image: The Journal of Nursing Scholarship, 26,* 47–51.

Raines, D. A. (1992). *An analysis of the values influencing neonatal nurses' perceptions and behaviors in selected ethical dilemmas* [CD-ROM]. Abstract from: SilverPlatter File: Dissertation Abstracts Item: 190003

Ramos, M. C. (1989). Some ethical implications of qualitative research. *Research in Nursing and Health, 12,* 57–63.

Rest, J. R. (1975). Longitudinal study of the Defining Issues Test of moral judgement: A strategy for analyzing developmental change. *Developmental Psychology, 11,* 738–748.

Rest, J. R. (1982). A psychologist looks at the teaching of ethics. *Hastings Center Report, 12*(1), 29–36.

Schank, M. J., & Weis, D. (1989). A study of values of baccalaureate nursing students and graduate nurses from a secular and a nonsecular program. *Journal of Professional Nursing, 5,* 17–22.

Schuldenfrei, P. D. (1990). *Moral development in licensed practical nurses enrolled in an associate degree program in nursing* [CDROM]. Abstract from: SilverPlatter File: Dissertation Abstracts Item: 129219

Sheer, B. L. (1989). *The relationships among socialization, empathy, autonomy, and unethical student behaviors in baccalaureate nursing students* [CD-ROM]. Abstract from: SilverPlatter File: Dissertation Abstracts Item: 127907

Shipps, T. B. (1988). *Truthtelling behavior of nurses: What nurses do when physicians deceive clients* [CD-ROM]. Abstract from: ProQuest File: Dissertation Abstracts Item: 8902914

Silva, M. C. (1990). *Ethical decision making in nursing administration.* Norwalk, CT: Appleton & Lange.

Smith, J. S. (1989). *Implications for values education in health care systems: An exploratory study of nurses in practice* [CD-ROM]. Abstract from: SilverPlatter File: Dissertation Abstracts Item: 125121

Soderberg, A., & Norberg, A. (1993). Intensive care: Situations of ethical difficulty. *Journal of Advanced Nursing, 18,* 2008–2014.

Stoll, S. J. (1989). *The relationship between perception of organizational climate and the quality of nurses' ethical decisions across four levels of educational preparation* [CD-ROM]. Abstract from: SilverPlatter File: Dissertation Abstracts Item: 129212

Stone, J. B. (1989). *An analysis of ethics instruction and the preparation of ethics educators in graduate nursing programs in the United States* [CD-ROM]. Abstract from: SilverPlatter File: Dissertation Abstracts Item: 118994

Supples, J. M. (1993). Self-regulation in the nursing profession: Response to substandard practice. *Nursing Outlook, 41,* 20–24.

Taylor, E. J., Ferrell, B. T., Grant, M., & Cheyney, L. (1993). Managing cancer pain at home: The decisions and ethical conflicts of patients, family caregivers, and homecare nurses. *Oncology Nursing Forum, 20,* 919–927.

Theis, E. C. (1988). Nursing students' perspectives of unethical teaching behaviors. *Journal of Nursing Education, 27,* 102–106.

Thurston, H. I., Flood, M. A., Shupe, I. S., & Gerald, K. B. (1989). Values held by nursing faculty and students in a university setting. *Journal of Professional Nursing, 5,* 199–207.

Turner, S. L. (1990). *An evaluation of the effectiveness of a guided design instructional package on ethical decision-making of senior nursing students* [CD-ROM]. Abstract from: SilverPlatter File: Dissertation Abstracts Item: 137390

Uden, G., Norberg, A., Lindseth, A., & Marhaug, V. (1992). Ethical reasoning in nurses' and physicians' stories about care episodes. *Journal of Advanced Nursing, 17,* 1028–1034.

Viens, D. C. (1992). *The moral reasoning of nurse practitioners* [CD-ROM]. Abstract from: SilverPlatter File: Dissertation Abstracts Item: 166791

Wehrwein, T. A. C. (1990). *Moral reasoning and ethical decision-making in beginning baccalaureate nursing students* [CD-ROM]. Abstract from: SilverPlatter File: Dissertation Abstracts Item: 147309

Weis, D., Schank, M. J., Eddy, D., & Elfrink, V. (1993). Professional values in baccalaureate education. *Journal of Professional Nursing, 9,* 336–342.

Wellard, S. (1992). The nature of dilemmas in dialysis nurse practice. *Journal of Advanced Nursing, 17,* 951–958.

Wiley, K., Heath, L., & Acklin, M. (1988). Care of AIDS patients: Student attitudes. *Nursing Outlook, 36,* 244–245.

Wilson, F. L. A. (1991). *The effects of age, gender and level of education on moral reasoning among registered nurses* [CD-ROM]. Abstract from: ProQuest File: Dissertation Abstracts Item: 9123653

Zalumas, J. C. (1989). *Critically ill and intensively monitored: Patient, nurse, and machine—the evolution of critical care nursing* [CD-ROM]. Abstract from: SilverPlatter File: Dissertation Abstracts Item: 119015

PART V

Other Research

Chapter 10

Nursing Research in Israel

HAVA GOLANDER
DEPARTMENT OF NURSING
TEL AVIV UNIVERSITY

TAMAR KRULIK
DEPARTMENT OF NURSING
TEL AVIV UNIVERSITY

CONTENTS

Recent years have witnessed an upsurge of review publications concerning the development of nursing research on several levels: national (Hopps, 1994; Lerheim, 1994; Van Swieten-Duyfjes & Grypdonck, 1994), continental (Tierney, 1994), and international (Bergman, 1990a, 1990b; Kim, 1994; Meleis, 1994). This chapter offers a review of Israeli nursing research during the past 35 years. Its purpose is to highlight basic processes and factors that have shaped nursing research in Israel and thus contribute to the international macro-analysis dialogue currently under way. National-level reviews are useful both for creating an international comparative data source and for instigating self-reflection and development. According to Cooper (1982) and Ganong (1987), the review constitutes primary research in itself, demanding systematic data selection and analysis. A national-level review, therefore, provides the possibility of bringing together, documenting, and classifying the accumulating body of research. It seeks to identify gaps and continuities, faults and successes, to point to new directions and set future agendas. The review provides a presentation of the discipline's development, and in doing this must come to terms with the widespread predicament among nursing scholars that in spite of its accumulated body of knowledge the discipline has not yet managed to present its successes to others, to market itself as an academic profession, or to break beyond its own professional and disciplinary boundaries. The academic voice of nursing is still muffled, and its impact on health policies has remained largely marginal (Gortner, 1980; Mathieson, 1994; Meleis, 1994; Styles, 1982; Tierney, 1993). A review of nursing's body of research is therefore of particular importance, especially in periods of accelerated change in health policies, as is the case today in many countries, including Israel.

DEVELOPMENT OF NURSING RESEARCH: ORGANIZING FRAMEWORKS

The organizational framework of this review of nursing research in Israel is based on two examples: first, the history of nursing research in the United States, which provided an excellent example of a national chronological development; and second, Bergman's (1990b) *Nursing Research for Nursing Practice*, which provided a useful example of comparative developmental perspective.

Whereas Florence Nightingale is usually considered the pioneer of nursing research, it is customary to mark the beginning of the research stage in nursing at 1952, when the journal *Nursing Research* was first published in the United States. In its 25th anniversary issue, *Nursing Research* published several review papers, among these the Gortner and Nahm (1977) article, which provided a clear account of the development of nursing research in the United States. According to the authors, early major investigations were commissioned by the profession to study needs and resources of nursing and nursing education. These studies were followed by investigations by graduates in nursing and related sciences. Research into nursing resources and services was a direct outgrowth of the nurse shortage in the 1950s and was commissioned by interested parties. Nurses continued to be the focus of research in the 1960s. Interest in nurses' traits and attributes, in educational opportunities, career mobility, and teaching methods was widespread. Practice-related research became the major focus of the 1970s and continues to prevail at present (Gortner, 1980).

The 1980s, as described by Polit and Hungler (1991), featured an important advancement, the establishment of the National Center for Nursing Research in 1986 at the National Institutes of Health. The American Nurses Association Commission on Nursing Research identified priorities that helped focus research on aspects of nursing practice. Several nursing specialty groups also developed research priorities within their domain of practice (Murphy & Freston, 1991). Research now opened to a growing interest in process-oriented studies employing qualitative research perspectives.

On the basis of reviews from 10 countries (Canada, Jamaica, Spain, Brazil, Israel, Sweden, the United States, Australia, New Zealand, and South Africa), Bergman (1990b) described a comparative model for the development of nursing research. The model is composed of five stages in relation to three interrelated aspects: content, method, and logistics or support systems.

Stage 1 focused on the "who" of nursing, or counting heads. Who were nurses? Where did they work? What were their demographic characteristics? Who were the applicants, and which candidates completed the educational program? The methods were largely descriptive. The major logistic priority was to recruit and prepare nurses to conduct research. The first generation of nursing doctorates were mostly administrators who had earned doctorates in education.

Stage 2 overlaps with the first, moving from "who" to "what." What were the nurses doing? The concern in this period was for optimum use of nursing time and energy. This was the model of choice, so it was necessary to differentiate between the type of care provided by the different levels of nursing personnel. Method 3 was primarily epidemiological with comparative designs. The increased scope of research highlighted the difficulties in funding research and underscored the need for developing a financial foundation for supporting research. Financial strategies for developing research included requests for government funding, foundation funding, and the construction of research units and institutes.

Stage 3 of the model was the "how" period, with a focus on clinical practice. At first, basic nursing skills were researched, and later, as clinical experts with advanced preparation entered the field, research expanded into more specialized subjects, such as cardiology, pediatrics, geriatrics, and oncology. The research emphasis was on how to improve the quality of nursing care. Methods in this phase included mainly quasi-experimental designs employed to compare alternative nursing procedures. This period was characterized by the logistics of dissemination, that is, a focus on the translation of findings into action. Journals devoted to nursing research flourished, and interest groups were founded.

Priorities of stage 4 showed a growing concern for social issues. Nurses researched the effects of social support at the individual, family, and community levels. Nurses became more involved with issues of health policy. For many researchers, grounded theory was the preferred method and was used for developing nursing theoretical frameworks.

Stage 5 presented a new emphasis: the meaning of nursing, values, and ethics. Researchers were seeking to define the quality of care and, more generally, quality of life. Phenomenological and anthropological approaches were used. Support systems for researchers were established and were spreading in the local, national, and international settings.

The model implies a historical progression, in which past priorities are still relevant today. The dilemma currently facing nursing researchers is whether to proceed systematically in the scientific elaboration of knowledge (Kim , 1987, 1994) or to emphasize the active involvement of nursing in shaping the social, political, and economic aspects of the health care system (Hopps, 1994; Meleis, 1994; Tierney, 1993).

Following is a brief overview to chart the general contours of the Israeli health care system, of which Israeli nursing is part and parcel. For an elaborate study of the politics, history, and sociology of the Israeli health care system, see Shuval's (1992) book.

ISRAELI HEALTH CARE SYSTEM: AN OVERVIEW

Because nursing and nursing research are an integral part of the health care system, it is essential to give a short background of the system in Israel. In 1948, when Israel was established, some organized health care services already existed. The British government had initiated a department of health and laid the infrastructure for what later became the Ministry of Health. Other health services were the various "sick funds," the largest of which was Kupat Holim, the sick fund of the General Federation of Laborers, whose ideology was based on an egalitarian health care system for all. To these one must add the voluntary services, the most notable being Hadassah.

Through the years, all these organizations have undergone various changes in the nature, size, and scope of care. Today 96% of Israel's population (5.5 million) is insured by one of the four sick funds that cover health care services in the public sector. The remaining 4% have sufficient income to meet their health care expenditures. Kupat Holim insures close to 70% of the population, which includes special coverage for the poor paid for by the Ministry of Health and provides the majority of primary care in some 1,300 community clinics in both urban and rural areas. The Ministry of Health maintains maternal and child clinics with overall responsibility for preventive care. Although community-based preventive and long-term care are developing at a steady pace, long-term care services are still insufficient to meet the rapidly growing needs of all age groups.

Payment for hospitalization is covered by the sick funds and is provided to the entire population in public hospitals owned by the Ministry of Health, Kupat Holim, and Hadassah. At present, issues such as increasing health care costs and expenditures, the aging of the population, the enormous influx of new immigrants, and changes in health care consumerism are confronting the health care system. As a result, major health care reforms are taking place. This includes the implementation of a mandatory health care law and the transformation of the main medical centers into corporations. These changes will force health care providers, especially nurses, to foresee and accommodate additional changes in services and education.

Important changes have taken place in education as well. The move from hospital-based diploma training to independent schools began in 1965 and progressed to the introduction of academic education in 1968, first as post-basic courses for registered nurses, followed by continuous academization of most schools of nursing. An important contribution to nursing higher education, especially to research, was the establishment of the master's degree program at Tel Aviv University in 1982. In recent years, nurses have been obtaining doctoral degrees in various fields in several universities in Israel.

Following is a review of the accumulation of nursing research in Israel. The development of research over time is examined following Bergman's model (1990b), according to three axes: content, methods, and logistics. We begin by describing our data sources for the review and conclude with several implications for the future.

METHOD OF REVIEW

Empirical data for this review are based on several sources. For the historical review of nursing research the revised edition of the compilation of nursing research in Israel was used (Bergman & Rottem, 1993), which lists published and unpublished research conducted from 1959 on. It is the most systematic and complete source of data regarding nursing research in Israel and first appeared in 1970 (and thereafter in 1972, 1980, 1985, 1987, 1989, 1992, and 1993). The first edition (1970) included 30 items; the last one (1993) had 332. Research is subsumed in the compilations under four categories: clinical, education, administrative, and social aspects (including opinions and views). The same categories were used to analyze the data for this review. The format of the anthologies, which includes the researcher's name, the framework of the research, and the year of publication, allowed for a secondary analysis of this material (see Table 10.1), leading to some general conclusions regarding the stages of research in Israel.

Table 10.1 Number of Nursing Research Projects Conducted in Israel According to Period and Research Domains

	Research Domains				
Period	Clinical	Administrative	Education	Social	Total
1960	—	—	1	—	1
1961–1970	5	8	16	7	36
1970–1980	22	18	20	19	79
1981–1990	48	32	22	33	135
1991–1993	26	24	20	11	81
Total	101	82	79	70	332

To widen, deepen, and verify the analysis, several complementary sources were used: master's theses and projects abstracts from the Master's Program in Nursing at Tel Aviv University, data taken from an evaluative study of the program's graduates (Golander, Bergman, Krulik, & Rottem, 1993), and relevant publications and personal interviews conducted with key informants and researchers.

HISTORICAL DEVELOPMENT OF NURSING RESEARCH IN ISRAEL

Israeli nursing research has changed over the years in both nature and scope (Bergman & Rottem, 1993). Table 10.1 shows the directions of growth in the scope of research and the change of research focus in the past 35 years. In what follows, the contents, methods and the logistics of study are described for each period.

The 1960s (1959–1970)

The first period of nursing research produced 37 studies, almost half in education (46%) and the rest in administration (22%), social (19%), and clinical (13%) aspects of nursing. In education, topics for research included: characteristics of nursing students and their teachers, factors contributing to completion of studies, preparation of students to professional life and follow-up surveys on nursing school graduates. In the administrative domain, the major concern was in work activities and shortage of nurses. Special mention should be made of the national study of nursing activities (Ben-Dov, 1966) initiated by the Ministry of Health and conducted by a neutral research institute. This study showed that about one third of nursing time was dedicated to nonnursing activities. Following this study, the number of nursing positions was increased. In the social domain, images of nurses were studied, as well as nurses' readiness to work in relatively novel areas such as geriatrics, family counseling, and care of new immigrants. Clinical research focused on health care needs in the community. A great deal of the research was conducted not by nurses nor with a nurse as a second investigator; nurses were the object of study for social scientists, on the one hand, and policy makers on the other. Twenty-five percent of the research (8 studies) was conducted by nurses as part of their master's degree program (6 studies) and doctoral degrees (2), taken in public health (5) and education (3). Master's degrees were given by Israeli universities, whereas doctorates were attained in the United States. Research subjects were dictated by the academic interests of the supervisors, who came from disciplines other than nursing, and by the researchers' fields of specialty. For most of this period, an academic framework for acquiring higher degrees in nursing was still nonexistent. Researchers were few: one researcher (Bergman) participated in 20% of the studies. The methods employed were usually the epidemiological survey and quantitative analyses.

The 1970s (1971–1980)

This period showed, for the first time, a relatively equal distribution among the four basic research domains: clinical (28%), education (25%), social aspects (24%), and administration (23%). Clinical research had varied its scope, spreading to additional health care sectors such as children's wards, internal wards, psychiatry, geriatrics, and home care of the chronically ill. Clinical researchers also began to study the effectiveness of various nursing interventions, such as patient education and satisfaction. Eighty-two percent of the clinical research was conducted as part of master's degree (16) and doctoral (2) studies; most of the students were the first graduates of the baccalaureate program of the Department of Nursing at Tel Aviv University, which was opened in 1968.

In the research domain of education, about 65% of the research was conducted by nurses studying for a master's (12) or doctoral (1) degree, mostly in schools of education. Social research also was primarily conducted by students (63%) as part of their master's (11) and doctoral (1) degrees, taken in one of the following departments: public health (8), criminology (2), psychology (1), and education (1). Research in the administrative domain was different in one respect; it was still the concern of state institutions such as the Ministry of Health and the Ministry of Labor and of institutes for health insurance. Only 2 of the 18 administrative studies were conducted solely by nurses as part of their theses in public health. Both studied patients' ratings of nursing services. As to the methods and logistics, most of the studies were surveys and simple quantitative research, for which nurses only rarely received funding.

The 1980s (1981–1990)

The 1980s produced 139 research projects, providing a 170% increase in the volume of research compared to the former period. Although education-related research was dominant in the first decade, the third period was dominated by clinical research (35.5%). Administration (24%) and social aspects (24%) remained stable, but education fell to 16% of all nursing research. The spectrum of research subjects continued to spread, and there was improvement in research methods with the introduction of qualitative methodology, clinical experimental designs, and historical research. Perhaps this could be attributed to the Master's Program in Nursing, which opened in 1982 in the Department of Nursing of Tel Aviv University, and produced in this period 59 theses, 43% of the whole nursing research conducted in that period. The opening of other academic nursing schools, such as Hadassah, at the Hebrew University in Jerusalem, and the Department of Nursing at the Ben Gurion University in Beer Shebah, clearly contributed to the scope and quality of research conducted mainly by faculty members. In the mid-1980s a research unit was established in the Department of Nursing of Tel Aviv University; its roles included counseling and support to students and faculty, as well as identifying possible sources of funding. There is no doubt that this unit gave a big thrust to the amount and quality of research.

In clinical research, new topics included self-care, stress and adjustment, disease and rehabilitation trajectories, family adjustment, and nurse-patient relations. Eighty percent of this research was conducted as part of master's degree (36) and doctoral degree (2, in the U.S.) studies. The domain of social aspects also has undergone a significant change. It moved from the study of nurses' opinions and images to the study of professional behavior, clinical decision making, and ethical dilemmas. Complex and sensitive issues, such as family adjustment to cancer, the meaning of life in nursing homes, and recurrent hospitalizations of the elderly, were studied for the first time. Fifty-seven percent of this social-aspects–related research was conducted as part of studies for higher degrees (19). For the first time, four nurses undertook doctoral studies in Israeli universities, in the fields of criminology, sociology, philosophy, and education. Research in the area of administration also gradually moved to the university. About 75% was now conducted by master's degree students, mostly in labor relations and, after 1985, in the Master's Program in Nursing. Typical administration-related subjects included nurses' stress and absence from work and nurses quitting work. Toward the end of this period, quality of care became a research topic. In the domain of education, new research topics included the behavior of students in specific care situations (e.g., terminal illness) and malpractice.

The 1990s (1991–1993)

The first 3 years of the fourth period produced 81 studies, on the basis of which it might be expected that nursing research would continue to be dominated by clinical studies conducted by nursing students in master's degree programs. The focus of research had moved to care of symptoms and pain, psychogeriatrics, quality of life, and quality of care. Administrative research was focused on job enrichment and the identification of organizational factors contributing to the quality of care. Educational research concerned itself with clinical instruction, acquired immunodeficiency syndrome (AIDS) prevention, and AIDS care. Social research continued to deal with sensitive matters such as sexuality and pressing ethical issues.

The 1990s show continuation of qualitative, quantitative, and historical studies. There is an increase in evaluative research in clinical interventions and teaching methods as well as studies that combine qualitative and quantitative methods.

Changes are also occurring within the health care services. Several large medical centers now have posts in which nurses can carry out epidemiological and quality assurance research. Funding is still scarce, although nurses occasionally receive grants from various institutions. The absence of a specific national fund for nursing research is sorely felt.

RESEARCH DISSEMINATION

Due to lack of appropriate venues for dissemination of nursing research, for years researchers had to use international journals and conferences to make their work known. Only in recent years has *The Nurse in Israel* (the main professional journal since 1948) begun to publish research articles. In the late 1980s, several interest groups started their own journals, for example, oncology and cardiology nursing, and from time to time also published research articles. It should be noted that none of the journals is refereed. Beginning in the 1970s, the Department of Nursing of Tel Aviv University began to bring out anthologies of research done by faculty and master's degree students on subjects such as nursing personnel, quality of care, and history.

Parallel to the journals, biannual national conferences gradually began to play a large role in spreading research findings. In the latest conference, held at the end of 1994, 60% of the papers presented were research-oriented.

Developments in nursing research have brought with them an urgent need to establish a high-quality refereed journal of nursing. Unfortunately, because universities value foreign publications, primarily for promotion, it may be some time before such a journal is launched.

FROM THE PAST INTO THE PRESENT: MAJOR TRENDS AND ACTIVITIES

Beyond the significant increase in the volume of research and the number of researchers ($N = 295$), there has been a considerable development in nursing research in Israel. The evolutionary trend in research content and methodology was similar to that in other countries. However, the logistics of building an infrastructure for research is lagging behind and requires immediate attention if nursing research is to continue its development. Two case studies are used to illustrate the unique research logistics characteristic of Israel. These are the national surveys of quality of care (Ron & Bar-Tal, 1993; Vin, Ron, & Bar-Tal, 1991) and the research groups of The Forum for Psychogeriatric Nursing.

The National Survey of Quality of Care

This survey was conducted in 13 Israeli general hospitals toward the end of the 1980s. It was initiated by the Nursing Department of the Ministry of Health in collaboration with researchers from the Department of Nursing of Tel Aviv University. The principal scientist of the Ministry of Health provided approximately U.S. $25,000 for funding. The research tool was a monitoring instrument developed by Goldstone, Ball, and Collier (1983) in Britain. Data collection included observations, nursing files, interviews with patients, and questionnaires. Data were collected by hospital nurses trained by the researchers. Discussing the findings of this survey is beyond the scope of this review (but see Ron & Bar-Tal, 1993; Vin, Ron, & Bar-Tal, 1991). It should be noted that each hospital received a copy of the survey's report and that teams were organized to seek solutions to the faults identified in the report. Far beyond its practical implications, the survey also had a multidimensional ripple effect: First, many hospitals allocated a position for a nurse responsible for quality control of the care given in the institution. Second, the intensive research effort and the involvement of a large number of nurses in it contributed to an internalization of the idea of nursing research and to a positive competition over quality of care among hospitals. In the latest national conference of nurses, in 1994, a large number of studies, conducted and presented by practicing nurses, showed a concern with improving nursing care. Third, the national survey provided the necessary data base for a number of theses and projects conducted within the Master's Program in the Department of Nursing, Tel Aviv University, and for other follow-up surveys (Ron, 1994).

In sum, the national survey is a positive example of a "top-down" process that introduced new goals, contents, and research experience for Israeli nurses. It opened a new era for research initiatives and collaborations between the academy and the service. Despite its importance and complicated nature, the research received only minimal funding. The nurses who collected the data did not receive payment. The hospitals and the university paid for the extra work time and for the statistical analysis. Previous social relations that existed among the nurses and the researchers, and the overall commitment to the research, contributed to its quick completion in 2 years with minimal funding.

Research Groups of the Forum for Psychogeriatric Nursing

In the beginning of the 1980s an interdisciplinary committee (Bergman & Golander, 1982; Bergman, Golander, Natan, Rabinowitz, & Ron, 1982) produced a general model for quality of care of the elderly. This model later served as the basis for a series of field studies initiated by Professor Bergman and her group in the Department of Nursing, Tel Aviv University. The studies were supported by a small grant from the Brookdale Institute for Gerontology. Researchers went out to the field, observing and interviewing elderly people at home and in nursing wards, their families, and the nurses. This led to the development of a conceptual model and a comprehensive research instrument for examining the quality of care in psychogeriatric units (Bergman & Gerstansky, 1987). The next stage was developing a project for testing this instrument, for which a small grant was provided by Eshel, a governmental body encouraging initiatives concerning services for the elderly. The project included meetings in six psychogeriatric institutions. Nurses who heard about the group's work asked to join it, and at the end of the year the group counted 50 nurses representing 20 institutions. In their final reports, the principal researchers claimed that the project had succeeded beyond their expectations (Bergman, Gerstansky, & Lindenbaum, 1991, 1992). The quality of care in the ward was significantly improved, the nurses' own professional image was increased, and the staff was encouraged to learn new ways of care and to experience, for the first time, guided research activity.

The project continued, and the Psychogeriatric Nursing Forum organized as a national interest group. It now comprises more than 15 active research groups conducting studies on the cutting edge of psychogeriatric nursing, particularly regarding dementia. Each research group has about five members from different institutions, plus a methodological consultant who is a teacher in the Department of Nursing, Tel Aviv University. Research topics address specific applied questions of practical and theoretical merit such as the following: When can bathing in the Jacuzzi serve as therapy for demented patients? How can dolls be used positively with demented patients? What is the reaction of demented patients to their mirror reflection? How can physical restraining of demented patients be kept to a minimum? And what types of social networks develop among demented patients? The methods used for such studies are extremely variable, ranging from experimental designs and case study analysis to participant observations, questionnaires, and interviews. Findings are presented in the wider meetings of the forum and published in professional journals.

In summary, research conducted within the forum tends to generate clusters of knowledge relevant to nursing of demented patients. The diversity in the background of participants created a fruitful basis for research. In terms of research logistics, the forum was not preplanned but rather "naturally occurred." One important development enabled by this natural process was a move from top-down projects to bottom-up studies. The number of participants in the research groups of the forum has increased continually, now reaching more than 100. In the absence of funding, the research activity is conducted on a voluntary basis. The price is that there is virtually no guiding long-term research policy. However, the forum activities had already proved their ability to change local policies and practices of nursing wards.

FUTURE TRENDS

Nursing research in Israel is currently at an important junction, created both by the imminent reforms in the Israeli health care system and by the lag in the development of research logistics. The development of Israeli nursing research in the past was largely abnormal. In regard to contents and methods, Israeli nursing research can be classified in the fifth, most advanced level according to Bergman's model (1990b), described above; in logistics, however, it still lags behind, in the second stage, which is the development of funding resources. Until now, the problem of funding was met with on-the-spot solutions, such as self-funding by researchers, absorption of costs by the workplace, voluntary work, and applications to general funding agencies. This abnormal situation cannot continue after the activation of health reforms. Hospitals are expected to become financial corporations and will not tolerate any devotion of time by nurses to external research projects. It seems that, at least during the first stage of the reform, all financial resources will be devoted to improving facilities and care, which may harm the development of nursing research.

Only a small number of elite researchers from two universities are responsible for the advances in nursing research in Israel. The increased number of researchers over the years is directly related to the increase in the number of master's and doctoral degree students. However, graduates with these higher degrees usually do not continue research activity. The follow-up survey conducted with graduates of the Master's Program in Nursing, Tel Aviv University, has shown that only 10% reported on some research involvement after their graduation. More encouraging is the finding that 43% expressed a wish to remain connected with the department's teachers through research (Golander et al., 1993). Most nurses in Israel have positive attitudes toward research (Ehrenfeld & Eckerling, 1991) and are interested in improving their work by using research findings. However, they do not perceive their organizational environment as encouraging and promoting such interests (Rachmani, 1994).

One of the weaknesses of the infrastructure for nursing research in Israel is the fact that organizations other than academe are not sufficiently involved in the development of research. The literature shows that in virtually every country education was the motivating force behind nursing research. Nonetheless, other bodies also participated in that task, such as the nurses' associations. In the United States, for example, there is a long tradition of governmental involvement in funding studies for higher degrees, academic programs, and research. The National Institute for Nursing Research, for instance, is responsible for supporting a cadre of researchers, managing research programs, and disseminating research reports. The establishment of this institute indicates the equal place given to nursing in relation to medical science. Federal funding enables nursing to avoid the "shotgun" studies that characterized the past and to focus on relevant issues and appropriate research designs (Hinshaw & Heinrich, 1990). The American Nurses Association Cabinet on Nursing Research (1985) also played a significant role in publishing opinions and reviews, setting research policies and priorities. In Britain, government offices have collaborated with professional organizations like the Royal College of Nursing (RCN) to support the development of research units, positions, and grants (Hopps, 1994). Similar facilities were created in Canada (Flaherty, 1990), Scandinavia (Lerheim, 1994), and South Africa (Searle, 1990). In developing countries, the World Health Organization supported the establishment of research institutes (Bergman, 1990a).

In Israel, however, there have been no governmental and/or professional bodies to support the construction of organizational facilities required for research. The call to establish such a research institute, issued by the Department of Nursing (Bergman, 1977, 1992), was left unanswered because there were no allies in the establishment. The Israeli Nursing Association (INA) did assemble a committee on research in 1967, but this committee allocated a minor role for itself. It limited itself to compiling nursing research projects conducted in Israel, promoting their publication, and identifying funding resources (Kirshenbaum-Galili, 1967). In practice, the INA did very little even in attaining these limited goals. Although the professional interest groups formed in Israel during the past 3 years (oncology, cardiology, psychiatry, surgery, and psychogeriatry) share a high level of awareness regarding the importance of research, these groups are too busy with their own process of consolidation and development to focus on research. The Nursing Department in the Ministry of Health is busy preparing for health reforms. In the light of this predicament, several future recommendations regarding logistics, contents, and method can be defined.

Logistics.   Until now, nursing research in Israel did not develop according to a predesigned plan but rather "occurred" (Bergman, 1977). The establishment of a proper infrastructure is now needed more than ever. Paradoxically, it is possible that the coming reforms in the health care system will produce the needed collaboration between nursing and medical sciences, as the latter shares the former's concerns regarding the future of research. Of high priority is the establishment of a government-based nursing research institute, which will concern itself with the following aims:

1. Set a national research policy and priorities for nursing research.
2. Initiate, encourage, coordinate, and manage long-term research in relevant fields.
3. Provide funding and research facilities for researchers through student scholarships and research grants.
4. Handle a complete and updated registry of nursing research in Israel.
5. Assemble relevant research literature, tools, and data, and promote the dissemination of original research among nurses through national and scientific publications.
6. Establish a library for nursing research or provide funding for existing libraries.
7. Develop and support research positions for nurses in the government, health institutes, and universities.
8. Promote disciplinary, interdisciplinary, and international research collaborations, including exchange of researchers.
9. Represent the interests of nursing research in the government and health institutes.
10. Collaborate with international research institutes.

Contents and Methods.   What are the recommended elements of future nursing research? Dutton and Crowe (1988) suggest 13 criteria for the assessment of research proposals, subsumed under the following categories:

1. Scientific merit (significance, potential, uniqueness).
2. Social benefit (improvement of the human condition and social understanding).
3. Programmatic concerns (institutional implications, international involvement).

Future research should direct itself to these aims. Scientific merit should be decided upon by the university; programmatic concerns, particularly critical health problems associated with the reforms, should be dealt with by the new research institute and researchers in the health organizations. As to social benefit, it is interesting to note that nursing research has not paid enough attention to exposing social problems and reflecting social heterogeneity. Nursing research will have to devote more attention, in the future, to issues of immigrants' adjustment, cultural differences, life in the shadow of war and terrorism, and the rehabilitation of young handicapped persons.

Bergman (1992) suggests a broad framework for determining research priorities on three levels, which she termed "ever-ever," "situational" and "never-never." The first group includes research that should be ongoing or periodic in all settings: quality of care, staffing, utilization of research, probing surveys, and seminal studies. The second category is related to a specific time, place, researcher, methods, or resources; for example, clinical research is needed today in regard to the old-old, the chronically ill, AIDS, and substance addiction. The never-never studies are those that carry little relevance for nursing, such as overreplicated studies.

The first two categories will evidently be important in the future. In addition, the field of evaluating nursing intervention should be far more developed. Pioneer studies are needed in the fields of medical technology and cost-benefit elements of informal care. In regard to methods, the use of clinical experimental designs and action research should be widened. Long-term and interdisciplinary research also should be encouraged. In retrospective, the 35 years of nursing research experience in Israel have produced a considerable amount of quality research, in spite of the limited resources at its disposal. The future challenge is to develop new research facilities and improve existing ones.

Reviewing the history of nursing research in Israel provided the opportunity to evaluate and reflect on its course, characteristics, strengths, and weaknesses. As a result of this process, action has been initiated. The deans and associates ($N = 13$) of the university schools of nursing agreed to form an interuniversity action group with the aim of establishing a national center for nursing research in Israel. The first step toward building the center would be to explore and determine national research priorities through the national interest groups. In addition, different models for the center's structure, affiliation, and budget are being considered.

REFERENCES

American Nurses Association Cabinet on Nursing Research. (1985). *Directions for nursing research toward the twenty-first century*. Kansas City, MO: Author.

Ben-Dov, N. (1966). *Nursing activities study*. Jerusalem: Ministry of Health.

Bergman, R. (1977). Overview of nursing research in Israel. *New Zealand Nursing Journal, 70*(9), 3–5.

Bergman, R. (1990a). All the world's a stage: The role of the international organization in nursing research. In R. Bergman (Ed.), *Nursing research for nursing practice* (pp. 1–10). London: Chapman and Hall.

Bergman, R. (1990b). Priorities in nursing research: Change and continuity. In R. Bergman (Ed.), *Nursing research for nursing practice* (pp. 195–203). London: Chapman and Hall.

Bergman, R. (1992). Setting priorities in nursing research. *Nursing RSA* [Republic of South Africa], *7*(4), 30–34.

Bergman, R., & Gerstansky, Y. (1987). *Development of an instrument to evaluate care in psychogeriatric units*. Tel Aviv: Tel Aviv University, Department of Nursing.

Bergman, R., Gerstansky, Y., & Lindenbaum, N. (1991). *Project to improve care in psychogeriatric units*. Tel Aviv: Eshel & Tel Aviv University, Department of Nursing.

Bergman, R., Gerstansky, Y., & Lindenbaum, N. (1992*). Project to improve care in psychogeriatric units*. Tel Aviv: Eshel & Tel Aviv University, Department of Nursing.

Bergman, R., & Golander, H. (1982). Evaluation of care for the aged: A multipurpose guide. *Journal of Advanced Nursing, 7*, 203–210.

Bergman, R., Golander, H., Natan, T., Rabinowitz, M., & Ron, A. (1982). *Quality of care in services for the elderly*. Jerusalem: Brookdale Institute of Gerontology and Adult Human Development in Israel (Hebrew).

Bergman, R., & Rottem, Z. (1993). *Research and studies on nursing in Israel*. Tel Aviv: Tel Aviv University, Department of Nursing.

Cooper, H. M. (1982). Scientific guidelines for conducting integrative research review. *Review of Educational Research, 52*, 291–302

Dutton, J., & Crowe, L. (1988). Views: Setting priorities among scientific initiatives. *American Scientist, 76*, 599–603.

Ehrenfeld, M., & Eckerling, S. (1991). Perception and attitudes of registered nurses to research: A comparison with a previous study. *Journal of Advanced Nursing, 16*, 224–232.

Flaherty, M. J. (1990). Nursing research: Cornerstone of nursing practice in Canada. In R. Bergman (Ed.), *Nursing research for nursing practice* (pp. 38–52). London: Chapman and Hall.

Ganong, L H. (1987). Integrative reviews of nursing research. *Research in Nursing and Health, 10,* 1–11.

Golander, H., Bergman, R., Krulik, T., & Rottem, Z. (1993*). Follow-up of master's degree graduates.* Tel Aviv: Tel Aviv University, Department of Nursing.

Goldstone, L. A., Ball, J. A., & Collier, M. M. (1983). *Monitor: An index of the quality of nursing care for medical and surgical wards* (2nd ed.). Newcastle upon Tyne: Polytechnic Products Ltd.

Gortner, S. R., & Nahm, H. (1977). An overview of nursing research in the United States. *Nursing Research, 26,* 10–33.

Gortner, S. R. (1980). Nursing research: Out of the past and into the future. *Nursing Research, 29,* 204–207.

Hinshaw, A. S., & Heinrich, J. (1990). New initiatives in nursing research: A national perspective. In R. Bergman (Ed.), *Nursing research for nursing practice* (pp. 20–37). London: Chapman and Hall.

Hopps, L. C. (1994). The development of research in nursing in the United Kingdom. *Journal of Clinical Nursing, 3,* 199–204

Kim, H. S. (1987). Structuring the nursing knowledge system: A typology of four domains. *Scholarly Inquiry for Nursing Practice: An International Journal, 1,* 99–110.

Kim, H. S. (1994). The need for knowledge in future nursing: Priorities in nursing research. In *Proceedings of the 7th Biennial Conference of the Workgroup of European Nurse-Researchers (WENR): The contribution of nursing research: Past–present–future* (Vol. 1, pp. 27–32). Oslo, Norway.

Kirshenbaum-Galili, H. (1967). The research committee for the development of nursing sections. *The Nurse in Israel, 64,* 10–38.

Lerheim, K. (1994). A perspective on Norwegian nursing research—past and present. In *Proceedinqs of the 7th Biennial Conference of the Workgroup of European Nurse-Researchers (WENR): The contribution of nursing research: Past–present–future* (Vol. 2, pp. 605–618). Oslo, Norway.

Mathieson, A. (1994). Nursing's new role in the future of research. *Nursing Standard, 8*(40), 19.

Meleis, A. I. (1994). A commitment for making a difference: Nursing care and research for the future. In *Proceedings of the 7th Biennial Conference of the Workgroup of European Nurse-Researchers (WENR): The contribution of nursing research: Past–present–future* (Vol. 1, pp. 47–56). Oslo, Norway.

Murphy, E., & Freston, M. S. (1991). An analysis of the theory-research linkage in published gerontology nursing studies, 1983–1989. *Advanced Nursing Science, 13*(4), 1–13.

Polit, D. F., & Hungler, B. P. (1991). *Nursing research: Principles and methods.* Philadelphia: Lippincott.

Rachmani, R. (1994). *Factors related to research utilization in nursing practice.* Unpublished master's thesis, Tel Aviv University, Tel Aviv.

Ron, R. (Ed.) (1994). *Quality assurance in nursing care.* Tel Aviv: Tel AvivUniversity, Department of Nursing (Hebrew).

Ron, R., & Bar-Tal, Y. (1993) . Quality nursing care survey, 1988–1990. *Quality Assurance in Health Care, 5*(1), 57–65.

Searle, C. (1990). Research as a modifier of the constraints in developing nursing practice in South Africa: An overview. In R. Bergman (Ed.), *Nursing research for nursing practice* (pp. 183–194). London: Chapman and Hall.

Shuval, J. (1992) . *Social dimension of help: The Israeli experience.* London: Praeger.

Styles, M. M. (1982). *On nursing: Toward a new endowment.* St. Louis: Mosby.

Tierney, A. J. (1993). Challenges for nursing research in an era dominated by health services reform and cost containment. *Clinical Nursing Research, 2,* 382–395.

Tierney, A. J. (1994). The development of nursing research in Europe. In *Proceedings of the 7th Biennial Conference of the Workgroup of European Nurse-Researchers (WENR): The contribution of nursing research: Past–present–future* (Vol. 3, pp. 159–185). Oslo, Norway.

Van Swieten-Duyfjes, E., & Grypdonck, M. (1994). Review of Dutch research on nursing of the chronically ill people, 1985–1993. *Proceedings of the 7th Biennial Conference of the Workgroup of European Nurse-Researchers (WENR): The contribution of nursing research: Past–present–future* (Vol. 2, pp. 973–981). Oslo, Norway.

Vin, Z., Ron, R., & Bar-Tal, Y. (1991). *Survey of quality of nursing care in public general hospitals in Israel.* Tel Aviv: Ministry of Health and Tel Aviv University, Department of Nursing (Hebrew).

Chapter 11

The Evolution of Nursing Research in Brazil

ISABEL AMÉLIA COSTA MENDES
COLLEGE OF NURSING
UNIVERSITY OF SÃO PAULO AT RIBEIRÃO PRETO

MARIA AUXILIADORA TREVIZAN
COLLEGE OF NURSING
UNIVERSITY OF SÃO PAULO AT RIBEIRÃO PRETO

CONTENTS

The purpose of this chapter is to analyze the course of nursing research in Brazil since the institutionalization of the profession in 1923. First, the necessity of nursing investigation and its awakening in the Brazilian context is presented. The authors then analyze the evolution of nursing research and identify the significant landmarks that initiated and stimulated its development. Subsequently, they present an overview of scholarly reviews of research in Brazil seeking a critical analysis of nursing research from the 1980s while emphasizing its meaning to diagnose the situation, to identify the obstacles and difficulties that surround the question of research, and to visualize expected goals, as well as a consciousness of the necessity of exchange among researchers, for expansion of Brazilian nursing knowledge. From the early development of nursing research in Brazil to the present, there has been significant progress, led by developments in the academic area. This review is limited to research described in dissertations and published in proceedings and journals. Finally, the challenges and necessities of nursing research in Brazil are presented.

THE NECESSITY FOR NURSING INVESTIGATION: AWAKENING IN THE BRAZILIAN CONTEXT

The expansion of health services and nursing services occurred as a consequence of industrialization, urbanization, and the rethinking of the concept of health by incorporating the social dimension. During the 1930s, 1940s, and 1950s, nursing changed into an essential element of the work force. Therefore, nurses' efforts were directed to the multiplication of services and to the formation of human resources, and research activity was relegated to a secondary position; consequently, it was fairly scarce. Di Lascio (1964) described this phase as follows:

> . . . nurses, overloaded with immediate problems caused by the new work fronts, did not have the opportunity or the stimulus to produce studies related to the profession, its functions and objectives. However, after the establishment of nursing services, nurses began to feel the necessity of high efficiency in the profession. Thus, the need for nursing scientific research arose. (pp. 201–202)

Nevertheless, during these decades, nurses generally were not prepared for research. The only national periodical specific to nursing was the *Brazilian Journal of Nursing,* created by the Brazilian Nursing Association (ABEn) in 1932, almost a decade after the creation of the first nursing school in Brazil. The themes of the articles published in the *Brazilian Journal of Nursing* until the middle of this century were basically (a) case studies; (b) nursing resources; (c) nursing practice, emphasizing patient care; (d) administration in nursing, focusing principally on the functions of the nurse; and (e) nursing education, placing great emphasis on nursing undergraduate courses, programs, and content, as well as on courses for nursing assistants, qualification of nursing professors, and the recognition of nursing schools. It is important to note that the articles did not originate from research but from personal experiences, tradition, authority, intuition, and loan (loan can be understood as a source of knowledge obtained from the appropriation and use of other disciplines' knowledge to orient nursing practice).

Circumstances led to the necessity for research in nursing. However, nurses did not receive formal research preparation in undergraduate courses, and they could not use the Brazilian Nursing Association journal to acquire this knowledge.

POINTS OF REFERENCE THAT UNCHAINED THE DEVELOPMENT OF RESEARCH

The Survey of Nursing Resources and Necessities (ABEn, 1980), concluded in 1958, is the first point of reference of scientific incorporation by Brazilian nursing. This study was motivated by the necessity for an inquiry about the situation of nursing in Brazil as well as by requests for information by international organizations, culminating in a solicitation from the Kellogg Foundation in 1957. Financed by the Rockefeller Foundation, the survey involved Brazilian nursing leaders from 1956 to 1958. The results, processes, and the methods used were presented at the International Didactic Seminar about Nursing Survey, promoted by the World Health Organization in July 1958 in Brazil.

The second point of reference of the scientific linkage of Brazilian nursing is a dissertation: the first nursing doctoral dissertation in Brazil and Latin America, presented by Glete de Alcântara (1963) of the University of São Paulo at Ribeirão Preto, College of Nursing, in 1963. This caused repercussions and various developments due to (a) the originality and level of the work and the importance of the author's theme, which was an analysis of the conditions surrounding the emergence of modern nursing as a profession and the obstacles to its expansion in the Brazilian society; (b) the author's leadership in the College of Nursing of Ribeirão Preto, which was founded and directed for 18 years by Glete de Alcântara, and the author's influence in the sphere of the Brazilian Nursing Association and its representation in international nursing.

The third point of reference, expressing the incorporation of research by nursing, was the 16th Brazilian Nursing Congress, held in 1964. The central theme was "Nursing and Research," following the suggestion of leaders of the Brazilian Nursing Association, who believed that nursing in Brazil had surpassed its infancy and adolescence and was moving into the adult phase. During this congress, Oliveira (1964) made favorable declarations about investment in research: direct or indirect participation in research and the importance of creating a new mentality in nursing, one in which professional affirmation will occur only as nurses search for a better delineation of nursing science, indispensable to the exercise of authentic and efficient practice. The development of this mentality belongs predominantly to undergraduate and graduate courses in Nursing Colleges. They have the responsibility for preparation of generalists and specialists, professionals capable of action in a world of change, who understand that changes are motivated by achievements in all branches of knowledge and technology.

Several specialists made contributions aimed at helping the participants acquire knowledge of the value of research in nursing. The land was cultivated and the seeds sowed. It was just a matter of waiting for the fermentation of ideas and the harvest of the first fruits. Indeed, Ferreira-Santos (1964) expressed her thoughts:

> I do not know if I have succeeded, with this work, in helping Brazilian nurses to feel what seems to me very clear: historical-social situations of the profession drove the nursing class to the necessity of research. Nurses are feeling the incentive for research—external motivation; however, they are not yet feeling the need for research—internal motivation. The steps I have pointed out as necessary to

form researchers will also be the ones that will develop the internal conscience, the truthful motivation for nursing research. (p. 288)

Therefore, the 16th Brazilian Nursing Congress (Schmarczek, 1982) recommended to the Brazilian Nursing Association:

(a) to stimulate the nursing colleges to prepare faculty members for research; (b) to promote courses and seminars about research methodology; and to the faculty members of the nursing colleges and the chiefs of nursing services: to utilize research in their work in order to obtain elements to evaluate it. (p. 71)

From 1964 until the end of the1970s, many nurses were motivated toward research, at least those linked to universities. Scientific production increased.

At the beginning of the decade of the 1970s, the fourth point of reference was manifested. It was possibly the most important and most profound in terms of its implications and the perspectives it could bring to the profession. The fourth point of reference is concerned with the entrance of nursing into the national system of graduate courses.

Since 1972, several master's degree courses were created at the most prominent nursing colleges of Brazil. In the late 1970s there were nine nursing master's degree courses at different points in Brazil, all of them having the principal objective of stimulating the development of research through the preparation of researchers.

The struggle of some nursing leaders to implement these programs, as well as the limited number of places in the courses, demonstrated and continue demonstrating that nurses linked to teaching feel a need for study and penetration of the area of research.

Thus, the requirements for academic qualifications for admission to and progress in a university career were driving forces in the development of nursing research and the preparation of nurse researchers in Brazil. Therefore, scientific production increased considerably. This enlargement caused two changes in the scenario of national nursing: (a) diversification of means of communication in the scientific community and (b) interest in the analysis of production.

In relation to the first change, the creation of other periodicals expresses the improvement of the production of knowledge. The *Brazilian Journal of Nursing,* launched in 1932, absorbed the production until 1966, when a gradual expansion of the demand for publications was verified. Seeking to fill this demand, another periodical was created in 1967; in the 1970s, four new periodicals; in the 1980s, another four; and in the 1990s, two. Looking at the periodicals, it is possible to infer that some states and some schools had the initiative to publish journals because of the large repressed demand for publication of articles. It is important to emphasize that, in spite of considerable efforts, some journals could not overcome the severe difficulties of lack of resources, principally financial, and became extinct. It is well known that the journals that succeeded in maintaining themselves also faced difficulties and needed to obtain resources from other sources. The journals that remain today are *Revista Brasileira de Enfermagem, Revista da Escola de Enfermagem da USP, Revista Paulista de Enfermagem, Revista Baiana de Enfermagem, Revista de Enfermagem da Universidade Estadual do Rio de Janeiro, Revista Enfoque, Revista Gaúcha de Enfermagem, Revista Latino-Americana de Enfermagem, Acta Paulista de Enfermagem,* and *Texto e Contexto: Enfermagem.* As another alternative, in 1977 the Brazilian Nursing Association created a new vehicle for the publication of official themes of Brazilian nursing congresses, the annals. This was an attempt to promote prompt dissemination of the core of discussions at congresses and at the same time to provide in the *Brazilian Journal of Nursing* publication of research presented as "Free Themes."

Referring to this second change—interest in the analysis of production— it is important to note that the more practice nurses acquired in research, the more questions they raised in relation to methodology, and for this reason they demanded more preparation for research. Because there were no nursing doctorate courses in Brazil, some researchers sought this study in other areas (Mendes, 1991).

In 1981, the University of São Paulo, through the nursing colleges of Ribeirão Preto and São Paulo, created the first nursing doctorate course in Brazil and in Latin America. The results indicate that nurses are demonstrating a better understanding of research methods and are aiming to study problems in light of theoretical ideas, according to Angerami and Mendes (1989). At present a total of six nursing doctorate courses have been created (see Table 11.1).

These courses receive students from all over Brazil. However, considering that 83% of them are concentrated in the southeast of Brazil and given the Brazilian territorial extension, there are some personal and professional obstacles to nurses who would like to move to the south and southeast of Brazil looking for a higher education. Therefore, the colleges of nursing are searching for alternatives to reduce the length of time students are absent from their original institutions. Faculty members from the University of São Paulo, College of Nursing, present the nursing doctorate programs of the University of São Paulo at the Nursing College of the Federal University of Minas Gerais. The Nursing Graduation Network (REPENSUL) was created in the south of Brazil; it was formed by six universities from three states of this region for the formation of human resources.

Another alternative was found by the University of São Paulo at Ribeirão Preto, College of Nursing, WHO Collaborating Center for Nursing Research Development, through agreements for the establishment of doctorate programs with the University of Concepción, Chile, and two federal universities from

Table 11.1   Nursing Doctorate Courses in Brazil According to University, Year, Concentration, Area, Region, and State

University	Year	Concentration Area	Region and State
University of São Paulo, College of Nursing College of Nursing at Ribeirão Preto	1981	Nursing doctoral level interinstitutional program	Southeast of Brazil, State of São Paulo
Paulista School of Medicine, Department of Nursing	1986	Maternal-child nursing	Southeast of Brazil, State of São Paulo
Federal University of Rio de Janeiro, "Ana Nery" College of Nursing	1989	Nursing in the Brazilian social context	Southeast of Brazil, State of Rio de Janeiro
University of São Paulo, College of Nursing	1990	Nursing	Southeast of Brazil, State of São Paulo
University of São Paulo, College of Nursing at Ribeirão Preto	1991	Fundamentals of nursing	Southeast of Brazil, State of São Paulo
Federal University of Santa Catarina, Department of Nursing	1992	Philosophy of nursing	South of Brazil, State of Santa Catarina

the northeast region of Brazil. These concentrated programs reduce the time of study away from the base institution by 50%. Faculty members associated with this agreement initiate research projects, present conferences, and give courses at the students' original institution.

Colleges of nursing are studying additional alternatives, looking for the better use of resources to answer the demand for courses, principally in the north, northeast, and central-west of Brazil. The scientific production derived from the graduate courses has, in general, acquired dimension and density, allowing the expansion of knowledge beyond the critical vision of professional practice.

With the remarkable events of the 1970s and 1980s concerning graduate courses and the products that were included in the fourth point of reference, progress emerged at the nursing association level, promoting a change in its structure through the creation of new organs and other attributes. The Center of Nursing Studies and Research (CEPEn) was created in July 1979 and is one of the new organs demarking the fifth point of reference of nursing research in Brazil.

As questions about research were discussed only among researchers linked to teaching at the graduate level and considering that there was no channel through which the subject could be widely discussed (as it was not an official theme of Brazilian nursing congresses since 1964), an increasing number of nurses manifested their need to participate in discussions about problems, facilities, limitations, and research guidelines, as well as to analyze the course that research was taking in nursing. These motives led the CEPEn to organize the first National Seminar on Nursing Research (1st SENPE), in November 1979. Since then, seven seminars have taken place with the following objectives:

- To know and to synthesize the participants' opinions about priority areas and difficulties of nursing research as well as their application to professional practice; to examine problems of common interest or become familiar with the progress in this field of research (ABEn, 1979).
- To evaluate the situation of graduate programs and their product: research; to determine problems in the areas of research; to evaluate the financial support from governmental organizations to nursing graduate programs and research; to establish perspectives of graduate-level nursing courses and research teaching in Brazil for the next 5 years (ABEn, 1982).
- To study alternatives of methodological interpretation of scientific knowledge and to analyze their utilization for nursing scientific production (ABEn, 1984).
- To analyze research trends and the nurse-researcher profile (ABEn, 1985).
- To stimulate the interest of nurse assistants for research (ABEn, 1988).
- To advance discussions about theoretical and methodological approaches in nursing research (ABEn, 1991).
- To discuss the dichotomy between nurses' work (assistant or teaching) and nursing research; to offer courses about research to nursing professionals; to understand the connections and specificities of different stages of nursing research in all regions of Brazil; to encourage the exchange and the definition of strategies for the realization of nursing research interregionally; to discuss innovative experiences of graduate programs and identify their viability to nursing (ABEn, 1994).

The Eighth National Seminar on Nursing Research will take place in July 1995 in Ribeirão Preto and will be organized by faculty members of the University of São Paulo at Ribeirão Preto College of Nursing. The faculty members of the nursing college of Ribeirão Preto performed a significant role in the establishment and development of the Center of Nursing Studies and

Research connected to the Brazilian Nursing Association, demonstrating their leadership, together with the association, in the sphere of research in the national context.

It is possible to conclude that the previous seminars had an impact on the nursing scientific community, which is continuing to reflect about the subject according to analysis of Brazilian nursing leaders, who are seeking the production of knowledge in the area. This is the focus of the next topic.

A CRITICAL ANALYSIS OF NURSING RESEARCH IN BRAZIL: FROM THE 1980S

A few years after the creation of the first master's degree courses, scientific production was evaluated by numerous studies (Almeida, Gomes, Ruffino, & Silva, 1981; Angerami & Almeida, 1982; Lopes, 1983; Mendes & Trevizan, 1983a, 1983b; Neves, 1982; Nogueira, 1982; Ribeiro, 1982; Trevizan, Mendes, Fávero, & Nacarato, 1981; Vieira, 1980). Among these, Mendes and Trevizan (1983a) affirmed that the development of nursing research occurred in an irregular way in the 10 years after the creation of the master's degree courses. They indicated four factors that promoted this situation: (a) the researcher did not get involved with the research consumers, (b) priorities for research were absent, (c) the researcher was not conscious of the importance of the establishment of research guidelines, and (d) the manner of using the scientific method in the research process was faulty. Considering the last factor, these authors tried to answer the question: Is the lack of application of the research results linked to the form of conducting the selected method for the production of this research? Analysis of this production showed that there was extensive use of the inductive process (89.5%) and only 10.4% using the deductive process with the fragmentation of these processes at some stage. This finding was sufficient for the conclusion that the studies analyzed did not yet represent the production of scientific information of this field of knowledge. Considering this study and in the light of the theory of Popper (1980), Trevizan and Mendes (1983) showed the possibility of expansion of nursing knowledge under the prism of conjecture and refutation and held that, depending on the rigor of classification of the scientific level of a body of knowledge, nursing can be considered as possessing prescientific knowledge.

Research by Almeida (1984, 1991), Neves and Gonçalves (1984), Souza (1988, 1991), Castellanos and Salum (1988), Elsen, Bub, and Athof (1991), Trevizan and Mendes (1991), Mendes (1991), and Cianciarullo and Salzano (1991) was based on the argument that the expansion of nursing knowledge has been a constant concern. These authors pointed out historical events demonstrating the inquietude of Brazilian nursing leaders about this subject, and they alerted the reader to the necessity of thinking about this theme, exploring and debating it so that it can reach a larger possible number of professionals in order to stimulate the resources coming from financial agencies through the understanding of the limitations and perspectives. Finally, they stimulated the reader to put the subject in doubt so that it can take shape and several solutions can be tried.

An analysis of underlying sources of nursing knowledge produced in the 1970s was carried out by Mendes and Trevizan (1983b). An epistemological analysis, based on the model of Bruyne, Herman, and Schoutheete (1982), verified that (a) in the instance of the *morphologic pole,* the 10 sources that most contributed to the analyzed publications were nursing (27.6%), medicine (19.6%), administration (10%), education (8.6%), psychology (7.7%), health policies (5.7%), sociology (5.2%), philosophy (5.2%), biological sciences (2%), economy and politics (0.9%); and (b) from the *theoretical pole* point of view, the bibliographical references evolved from the principal sources of medicine, administration, and education. Three tendencies emerged from this analysis: first, constant technical information demonstrating the functionalism of nursing knowledge; second, concern about human resources formation; and third, in the end of the 1970s a concern related to the search to frame nursing in the area of human and social sciences, as these sciences supply a vein to socialization and social mutation. As to the *epistemologic pole,* Mendes and Trevizan (1983b) found that nursing knowledge was conditioned to attitudes of nurses' perception about their own world and to the information they received. Therefore, since the 1970s the analyzed articles showed nurses' independence of being simply executors of medical orders, characteristic of prior decades. The authors affirm that, epistemologically, it was an important improvement for nursing to stop searching for its validity and knowledge sources in other sciences. Nursing already possesses a sufficient amount of bibliographical sources to stimulate its own knowledge development and has the technical resources to validate it.

After a general approach to the question of research, researchers began to analyze the produced knowledge in the nursing specialities from the second half of the 1980s. Thus, in the area of maternal-infant nursing, Rocha, Silva, and Alessi (1984) characterized the majority of the studies (84.6%) as descriptive and 7.7% as analytical-ideological. According to these authors, most of the analyzed studies did not present a logical structure and did not show their theoretical-methodological linkages. They also concluded that "the articles do not mention the important question of the existence of different historical forms of articulation between nursing social practice and the society" (p. 188). Cozzupoli and Garcia (1985) reported a retrospective analysis and the perspectives of research in the area of maternal-infant nursing in Brazil and internationally, confirming the conclusions of general studies on nursing research in Brazil.

Bonilha, Horta, and Ribeiro (1987) analyzed the modalities of research in the area of pediatric nursing conducted in order to obtain academic degrees, from 1975 to 1985, in Brazil. They concluded that investigations on nursing care were predominant, most research followed the descriptive-analytical approach, and the qualitative method was hardly used. Rocha, Scochi, and Lima (1993) aimed at understanding knowledge in the area of pediatric nursing in Brazil through bibliographical references, whose titles about child assistance were classified according to prescriptive and analytical orientation. They considered that

> the analytical texts establish a new perspective to nursing in the complex universe of the health process of work, a perspective to diversify nursing care, assisting the clientele and establishing new ways of visualizing in the same client other necessities. The prescriptive texts elaborated technical procedures to orient the work, but they only reproduce the knowledge on biology, physiology and pathology that orients individualized clinical medicine. (pp. 88–89)

Arantes (1985), studying the area of psychiatric nursing, considered the production restricted and based on problem raising. After that, Stefanelli, Fukuda, Rolim, and Arantes (1987) emphasized themes in the area of psychiatric nursing, aiming at stimulating nurses to incorporate in their practice knowledge from these investigations. Among these authors' conclusions, it is important to consider the nurses' suggestion of disclosing the nursing research results among the practitioner nurses.

In the area of medical-surgical nursing, Koizumi, Takahashi, and Miyadahira (1985) concluded that studies are based on the biological area as well as being characterized as descriptive research.

Nogueira (1985) indicated that in the area of community nursing 71.4% of research projects were directed to nursing care; 14.3%, to services administration; 12.5%, to teaching; and 1.8%, to research. The author reported that the majority of studies in the area of community nursing care are related to the identification of the clientele's needs.

Moriya, Pereira, and Gir (1991) did a retrospective study and an analysis of research conducted by nurses about hospital infection. The authors observed the prevalence of research related to technical procedures, followed by epidemiological investigations and research on the performance of the commissions of hospital infection control.

Ruffino, Freitas, and Casagrande (1985) emphasized that nursing education was an important area of the investigations published in Brazilian nursing congresses and in the *Brazilian Journal of Nursing* from 1947 to 1981. However, they pointed out the necessity of in-depth studies in this area, taking into consideration the desirable scientific development of educational research as well as nursing research.

The results of a study conducted by Enoki, Ferraz, Carvalho, and Marziale (1987) presented communication as the essence of patient-nurse interaction in 15.15% of the analyzed articles and reported the need for more research in this area.

Concomitantly, other groups dedicated their studies to the nurse-researcher profile, the researcher's position in regard to the research results, and ethics in nursing research. Several such studies were conducted by Sena (1985), Lemos (1985), Gonçalves (1985), Rocha (1985), Souza (1985), and Gelain (1985). These articles mainly focused on nurse-researcher qualities, abilities, and values.

At the same time, some authors alerted the scientific community to the importance and necessity of communication of research results as a strategic step to their utilization in practice (Angerami, 1994; Castro, Miranda, Rodrigues, & Lima, 1985; Lopes, 1993; Mendes, 1991, 1993; Mendes & Trevizan, 1990). These authors emphasized the stage of knowledge presentation as part of the research process, questions on strategies for knowledge publication, communication patterns, leadership skills in managing projects, networks, and the creation and administration of means of publication.

Almeida (1985), Boemer (1985, 1994), Pelá (1985), Laganá (1989), Stefanelli, Salzano, and Oguisso (1990), and Martins, Boemer, and Ferraz (1990) considered questions about methodological alternatives, and Rocha and Silva (1987) analyzed the philosophical and ideological guidelines of nursing research in Brazil. These authors recommended an improvement in nursing analysis. They also concluded that there is a remarkable influence of positivism in dissertations and theses produced by nurses in Brazil, and they pointed out that "there is an emergent tendency of alternative proposals aiming at finding theoretical principles in other sources, as in the dialectic and phenomenology" (Rocha & Silva, 1987, p. 220).

These evaluations have been positive forces in promoting nursing development as they advocate the visualization of scientific balance and the diagnosis of points of fragility, as well as the search for ways and actions that can reduce difficulties in expanding nursing knowledge.

FINAL CONSIDERATIONS

The authors directed efforts to demonstrate the situation of nursing research, showing the causative landmarks in its development in the Brazilian context and delineating the state of art in terms of a critical view of authors interested in contributing to the expansion of nursing knowledge.

It is important to emphasize the decisive role performed by graduate programs in the scientific progress obtained. It is consensually recognized that the primary force of the history of nursing research in Brazil is the emergence, evolution, and production of graduate courses offering dynamic contributions to nursing and nurses in Brazil.

The analysis and review contained in this study allows the reader to verify that at the beginning of the 1980s studies about the development of nursing research in Brazil were initiated and that they included methodologies, thematics, tendencies, underlying sources, lacunas, and privileged lines.

The seminars on research have influenced and stimulated reflection about nursing through a scientific view validated by research. These events favor the analyses of graduate courses. Several specific events with the same objectives have been conducted by the universities that offer these courses and have been sponsored by CAPES Foundation, an agency that coordinates and evaluates graduate education in Brazil in all areas of knowledge. In these meetings, nurse leaders have the mission of evaluating the graduate courses and promoting an exchange among the nine master's degree courses and six doctoral courses in Brazil.

Therefore, it is possible to affirm that research is consolidated in the Brazilian nursing university sphere; the expansion caused by the graduate courses, the leaders and, nursing association actions, through the CEPEn, were decisive to the establishment of ideas, to the commencement of nuclei organizations, and to the promotion of a technical-scientific exchange among nurses in Brazil, beginning an international exchange.

Cianciarullo and Salzano (1990) described the important role of financing agencies for nursing research in Brazil, as these agencies support the development of research projects and finance graduate courses. On the other hand, they note that research on nursing care is not developed to the same extent as research in the academic area. Cianciarullo and Salzano affirm that "the distance maintained by practicing nurses from research constitutes a paradox for those who study research-based practice, seeking new forms or ways of performing and understanding the essentials of nursing" (p. 141).

Although research is not consolidated in the area of nursing care, there are efforts for its consolidation. Among them, there is the effort to encourage future nurses to acquire (a) a new mentality, (b) the custom of facing themes, organizing thought, and treating problems, (c) the capacity to argue based on literature references, and (d) interest and devotion to seeking coherent and consistent conclusions. Therefore, there is hope that future nurses in the care area will present a new profile and behavior directed by and for research, through a profound interaction with nurse-researchers linked to the academic area.

In spite of the difficulties, it is possible to affirm that in the 1990s the necessity for and importance of research are incorporated in the collective subconscious of nurses in Brazil. Although it is recognized that Brazilian nurses, especially in the academic area, are demonstrating competence in the trajectory of nursing scientific development, there is awareness that there are still limitations. It is important to emphasize that the efforts and enterprises need to come from groups, not individuals. As Mendes (1991) affirmed, the technical-scientific and financial vitalization will occur when nurses are producing in nuclei, groups, or big projects; then the research product will have a higher impact on Brazilian nursing.

Another challenge deserves attention and effort: the incisive investment in exchanges with developed centers to create collaborative projects and innovations to promote excellence in undergraduate and graduate teaching and research. The participation in postdoctoral courses and in short-term programs, manuscript publication in international journals, and the development of integrated projects are goals to pursue.

The necessity of exchange is incontestable; in a world more and more interdependent, countries necessarily need to relate to each other. In the context of interdependence, nursing at a world level must act in a spirit of collaboration that can be understood as an investment. If the actual tendency is globalization, nurses from several countries must act with this spirit, especially in the communication sphere. Then, through nursing journals and other means, nurses can look for a global integration with the consumption of produced knowledge.

REFERENCES

ABEn–Brazilian Nursing Association. (1979). *Relatório do Seminário Nacional de Pesquisa em Enfermagem* [Report of the National Seminar on Nursing Research]. Ribeirão Preto, Brazil: Universidade de São Paulo.

ABEn–Brazilian Nursing Association. (1980). *Relatório final do Levantamento de Recursos e Necessidades de Enfermagem no Brasil—1956/1958* [Final report of the Survey of Nursing Resources and Necessities in Brazil—1956/1958]. Brasília, Brazil: ABEn.

ABEn–Brazilian Nursing Association. (1982). *Relatório do Segundo Seminário Nacional sobre o Ensino de Pós-Graduaçao e Pesquisa em Enfermagem* [Report of the Second National Seminar on Graduate Teaching and Nursing Research]. Brasília, Brazil: CNPq-Conselho Nacional de Desenvolvimento Científico e Tecnológico.

ABEn–Brazilian Nursing Association. (1984). *Anais do III Seminário Nacional de Pesquisa em Enfermagem* [Annals of the Third National Seminar on Nursing Research]. Florianópolis, Brazil: Universidade Federal de Santa Catarina.

ABEn–Brazilian Nursing Association. (1985). *Anais do IV Seminário Nacional de Pesquisa em Enfermagem* [Annals of the Fourth National Seminar on Nursing Research]. São Paulo, Brazil: Universidade de São Paulo.

ABEn–Brazilian Nursing Association. (1988). *Anais do V Seminário Nacional de Pesquisa em Enfermagem* [Annals of the Fifth National Seminar on Nursing Research]. Belo Horizonte, Brazil: Universidade Federal de Minas Gerais.

ABEn–Brazilian Nursing Association. (1991). *Anais do VI Seminário Nacional de Pesquisa em Enfermagem* [Annals of the Sixth National Seminar on Nursing Research]. Rio de Janeiro, Brazil: Palmar Gráfica e Editora.

ABEn–Brazilian Nursing Association. (1994). *Anais do VII Seminário Nacional de Pesquisa em Enfermagem* [Annals of the Seventh National Seminar on Nursing Research]. Fortaleza, Brazil: Universidade Federal do Ceará.

Alcântara, G. (1963). *A enfermagem moderna como categoria profissional: Obstáculos a sua expansão na sociedade Brasileira* [Modern nursing as a professional category: Obstacles to its expansion in Brazilian society]. Unpublished doctoral dissertation, Universidade de São Paulo, Ribeirão Preto, Brazil.

Almeida, M. C. P. (1984). A construção do saber na enfermagem: Evolução histórica [The construction of nursing knowledge: Historical evolution]. In *Anais do III Seminário Nacional de Pesquisa em Enfermagem* (pp. 58–77). Florianópolis, Brazil: Universidade Federal de Santa Catarina.

Almeida, M. C. P. (1985). O materialismo histórico na pesquisa em enfermagem [Historical materialism in nursing research]. In *Anais do IV Seminário Nacional de Pesquisa em Enfermagem* (pp. 83–89). São Paulo, Brazil: ABEn.

Almeida, M. C. P. (1991). A pesquisa como parte do processo de trabalho do enfermeiro [Research is a part of the process of nurse's work]. In *Anais do Vl Seminário Nacional de Pesquisa em Enfermagem* (pp. 53–58). Rio de Janeiro, Brazil: Palmar Gráfica e Editora.

Almeida, M. C. P., Gomes, D. L. S., Ruffino, M. C., & Silva, G. B. (1981). A produção do conhecimento na pós-graduação em enfermagen no Brasil [Knowledge production in nursing graduate courses in Brazil]. In *Anais do XXXIII Congresso Brasileiro de Enfermagem* (pp. 119–126). Manaus, Brazil: ABEn.

Angerami, E. L. S. (1994). Para que serve a divulgação científica [The function of scientific divulgation]. *Revista Latino-Americana de Enfermagem, 2,* 1–2.

Angerami, E. L. S. & Almeida, M. C. P. (1982)). Divulgação do conheciment científico produzido na enfermagem [Divulgation of scientific knowledge produced in nursing]. In *Relatório do II Seminário Nacional sobre Ensino de Pós-Graduação e Pesquisa em Enfermagem: Avaliação e perspectiva* (pp. 108–127). Brasília, Brazil: CNPg.

Angerami, E. L. S., & Mendes, I. A. C. (1989). Marco teórico das investigações em enfermagem: Sua relação com as teorias de enfermagem [The theoretical boundaries of nursing investigations: Their relationship with nursing theories]. *Revista Gaúcha de Enfermagem, 10,* 20–24.

Arantes, E. C. (1985). Pesquisa em enfermagem psiquiátrica [Research in the area of psychiatric nursing]. In *Anais do IV Seminário Nacional de Pesquisa em Enfermagem* (pp. 42–44). São Paulo, Brazil: Unversidade de São Paulo.

Boemer, M. R. (1994). A condição de estudos segundo a metodologia de investigação fenomenológica [The conditions of study according to the methodology of phenomenologic investigation]. *Revista Latino-Americana de Enfermagem, 2,* 83–94.

Boemer, M. R. (1985). A fenomenologia na pesquisa em enfermagem [Phenomenology in nursing research]. In *Anais do IV Seminário Nacional de Pesquisa em Enfermagem* (pp. 90–94). São Paulo, Brazil: Unversidade de São Paulo.

Bonilha, A. L., Horta, A. L. M., & Ribeiro, M. O. (1987). Pesquisa em enfermagem pediátrica [Research in pediatric nursing]. *Revista da Escola de Enfermagem da USP, 21,* 117–134.

Bruyne, P., Herman, J., & Schoutheete, M. (1982). *Dinâmica da pesquisa em ciências sociais—Os pólos da prática metodológica* [Dynamics of research in social sciences: Poles of methodological practice]. Rio de Janeiro, Brazil: Francisco Alves.

Castellanos, B. E. P., & Salum, M. J. L. (1988). A relação entre a pesquisa e a prática em enfermagem no setor da saúde: Reflexões e experiências de enfermeiros do campo num trabalho de pesquisa participante [The relation between nursing research and practice in the health sector: Reflections and experiences of country nurses in a study of participant research]. In *Anais do V Seminário Nacional de Pesquisa em Enfermagem* (pp. 41–65). Belo Horizonte, Brazil: Universidade Federal de Minas Gerais.

Castro, I. B., Miranda, C. M. L., Rodrigues, A. P. S., Lima, M. J. (1985). Dificuldades na incorporação de resultados de pesquisa na prática de enfermagem [Difficulties of the incorporation of the nursing results in nursing practice]. In *Anais do IV Seminario Nacional de Pesquisa em Enfermagem* (pp. 193–242). São Paulo, Brazil: Unversidade de São Paulo.

Cianciarullo, T. I., & Salzano, S. D. T. (1990). Nursing and nursing research in Brazil. In *Nursing research worldwide: Report of the Task Force on International Nursing Research, International Council of Nurses* (pp. 139–149). Geneva, Switzerland: International Council of Nurses.

Cianciarullo, T. I., & Salzano, S. D. T. (1991). A enfermagem e a pesquisa no Brasil [Nursing and research in Brazil]. *Revista da Escola de Enfermagem da USP, 25*, 195–215.

Cozzupoli, C. A., & Garcia, T. J. M. (1985). Pesquisa em enfermagem materno-infantil [Research in the area of maternal-infant nursing]. In *Anais do IV Seminário Nacional de Pesquisa em Enfermagem* (pp. 31–41). São Paulo, Brazil: Unversidade de São Paulo.

Di Lascio, C. M. D. S. (1964). Enfermagem e pesquisa: Apresentação [Nursing and research: Presentation]. *Revista Brasileira de Enfermagem, 17*, 201–216.

Elsen, I., Bub, L. I. R., & Athof, C. R. (1991). A pesquisa como atividade inerente ao processo de trabalho do enfermeiro [Research as an inherent activity of the nurse's work]. In *Anais do VI Seminário Nacional de Pesquisa em Enfermagem* (pp. 59–66). Rio de Janeiro, Brazil: Palmar Gráfica e Editora.

Enoki, H., Ferraz, A. E. P., Carvalho, E. C., & Marziale, M. H. P. (1987). A produção cientifica da comunicação em enfermagem [Scientific production about nursing communication]. *Revista Brasileira de Enfermagem, 40*, 34–37.

Ferreira-Santos, C. A. (1964). Pesquisa: Responsabilidade nova das escolas de enfermagem [Research: A new responsibility of nursing schools]. *Revista Brasileira de Enfermagem, 17*, 278–290.

Gelain, I. (1985). A influência da pesquisa em enfermagem na modificação do enfoque de valores éticos [The influence of nursing research on the change of focus of ethic values]. In *Anais do IV Seminário Nacional de Pesquisa em Enfermagem* (pp. 138–142). São Paulo, Brazil: Universidade de São Paulo.

Gonçalves, L. H. T. (1985). Relacionamento orientador-orientando [Advisor-student relationship]. In *Anais do IV Seminário Nacional de Pesquisa em Enfermagem* (pp. 107–117). São Paulo, Brazil: Unversidade de São Paulo.

Koizumi, M. S., Takahashi, E. I. U., & Miyadahira, A. M. K. (1985) Pesquisa em enfermagem médico-cirúrgica. [Research in the area of medical-surgical nursing]. In *Anais do IV Seminário Nacional de Pesquisa em Enfermagem* (pp. 60–77). São Paulo, Brazil: Unversidade de São Paulo.

Laganá, M. T. C. (1989). A pesquisa qualitativa: Sistematização de temas geradores e técnicas de grupo [Qualitative research: Systematization of generator themes and group technics]. *Revista da Escola de Enfermagem da USP, 23,* 153–161.

Lemos, M. J. A. (1985). Conhecimento que o enfermeiro deve possuir para se iniciar como pesquisador [Knowledge that a nurse must have to be initiated as a researcher]. In *Anais do IV Seminário Nacional de Pesquisa em Enfermagem* (pp. 118–126). São Paulo, Brazil: Unversidade de São Paulo.

Lopes, C. M. (1983). *A produção dos enfermeiros assistenciais em relação a pesquisa em enfermagem num município paulista* [The production of care nurses in relation to nursing research in a municipality of the state of São Paulo]. Unpublished master's thesis. Universidade de São Paulo, Ribeirão Preto, Brazil.

Lopes, C. M. (1993). *Aplicaçao dos resultados de pesquisa na prática de enfermagem* [Application of research results in nursing practice]. São Paulo, Brazil: Savier.

Martins, J., Boemer, M. R., & Ferraz, C. A. (1990). A fenomenologia como alternativa metodológica para pesquisa: Algumas considerações [Phenomenology as a methodological alternative to research: Some considerations]. *Revista da Escola de Enfermagem da USP, 24,* 39–147.

Mendes, I. A. C. (1991). *Pesquisa em enfermagem. Impacto na prática.* [Nursing research. Impact on the practice]. São Paulo, Brazil: Editora da Universidade de São Paulo.

Mendes, I. A. C. (1993). Carta ao Leitor [Letter to the reader]. *Revista Latino-Americana de Enfermagem,* 1 7–8.

Mendes, I. A. C., & Trevizan, M. A. (1983a). Acerca da utilização do método científico nas pesquisas de enfermagem [Utilization of the scientific method in nursing research]. *Revista Brasileira de Enfermagem, 36,* 13–19.

Mendes, I. A. C., & Trevizan, M. A. (1983b). As fontes do conhecimento e as tendências subjacentes nos artigos publicados na Revista Brasileira de Enfermagem de 1970 a 1981 [The sources of knowledge and the subjacent tendencies of the articles published in the *Brazilian Journal of Nursing* from 1970 to 1981]. *Revista Brasileira de Enfermagem, 36,* 154–163.

Mendes, I. A. C., & Trevizan, M. A. (1990). Comunicação do conhecimento. Questões, barreiras e opções [Communication of knowledge: Questions, obtacles and options]. In *Anais do II Simpósio Brasileiro de Comunicação em Enfermagem* (pp. 107–120). Ribeirão Preto, Brazil: Unversidade de São Paulo.

Moriya, T. M., Pereira, M. S., & Gir, E. (1991). Pesquisas, conferências e artigos em infecçao hospitalar: Aspectos abordados pelos enfermeiros [Research, conferences and articles on hospital infection: Nurse's approaches]. *Revista da Escola de Enfermagem da USP, 25,* 29–40.

Neves, E. P. (1982). Vazios do conhecimento e sugestões de temáticas relevantes na área da enfermagem [Emptiness of knowledge and suggestions of important thematics to nursing]. In *Relatório do II Seminário Nacional sobre Ensino de Pós-Graduação e Pesquisa em Enfermagem: Avaliação e perspectiva* (pp. 50–72). Brasilia, Brazil: CNPg.

Neves, E. P., & Gonçalves, L. H. T. (1984). As questões do marco teórico nas pesquisas de enfermagem [The questions about theoretical marks in nursing research]. In *Anais do III Seminário Nacional de Pesquisa em Enfermagem* (pp. 210–229). Florianópolis, Brazil: Unversidade Federal de Santa Catarina.

Nogueira, M. J. C. (1982). A pesquisa em enfermagem no Brasil: Retrospectiva histórica [Nursing research in Brazil: Historical retrospective]. In *Relatório do II Seminário*

Nacional sobre o Ensino de Pós-Graduação em Enfermagem-Avaliação e perspectiva. (pp. 25–38). Brasilia, Brazil:CNPg.

Nogueira, M. J. C. (1985). Pesquisa em enfermagem comunitária [Research in the area of community nursing]. In *Anais do IV Seminário Nacional de Pesquisa em Enfermagem* (pp. 45–59). São Paulo, Brazil: Unversidade de São Paulo.

Oliveira, M. I. R. (1964). Enfermagem e pesquisa: Importância e significação [Nursing and research: Importance and meaning]. *Revista Brasileira de Enfermagem, 17,* 206–216.

Pelá, T. R. (1985). Utilização de alternativas metodológicas na pesquisa em enfermagem [Utilization of methodological alternatives in nursing research]. In *Anais do IV Seminário Nacional de Pesquisa em Enfermagem* (pp. 78–82). São Paulo, Brazil: Universidade de São Paulo.

Popper, K. R. (1980). *Conjecturas e refutações* [Cunjectures and refutations]. Brasília, Brazil: Editora da Universidade de Brasília.

Ribeiro, C. M. (1982). Perspectivas da pesquisa em enfermagem [Perspectives of nursing research]. In *Relatório do II Seminário sobre Ensino de Pós-Graduação e Pesquisa em Enfermagem: Avaliação e perspectiva* (pp. 73–81). Brasília, Brazil: CNPg.

Rocha, M. L. Q. (1985). Reflexões sobre a posição do pesquisador e da comunidade frente aos resultados da pesquisa em enfermagem [Reflection about the position of the researcher and the community facing the results of nursing research]. In *Anais do IV Seminário Nacional de Pesquisa em Enfermagem* (pp. 143–151). São Paulo, Brazil: Unversidade de São Paulo.

Rocha, S. M. M., Scochi, C. G. S., Lima, R. A. G. (1993). 0 conhecimento em enfermagem pediátrica: Livros editados no Brasil de 1916 a 1988 [Knowledge in pediatric nursing: Books published in Brazil from 1916 to 1988]. *Revista Latino-Americana Enfermagem, 2,* 77–91.

Rocha, S. M. M., & Silva, G. B. (1987). Linhas filosóficas e ideológicas na pesquisa em enfermagem no Brasil [Philosophic and ideologic lines of nursing research in Brazil]. *Revista Brasileira de Enfermagem, 40,* 214–221.

Rocha, S. M. M., Silva, G. B., & Alessi, N. T. (1984). Características do saber da enfermagem profissional na área materno:infantil: Análise do seu discurso [Characteristics of professional nursing knowledge in the maternal-infant area: Analysis of its discourse]. In *Anais do III Seminário Nacional de Pesquisa em Enfermagem* (pp. 172–195). Florianópolis, Brazil: Unversidade Federal de Santa Catarina.

Ruffino, M. C., Freitas, D. M. V., & Casagrande, L. D. R. (1985). Retrospectiva das publicações realizadas sobre educação em enfermagem: 1947–1981 [Retrospective of the publications on nursing education: 1947–1981]. *Revista Brasileira de Enfermagem, 38,* 245–256.

Schmarczek, M. (1982). 33 *anos do Congresso Brasileiro de Enfermagem: Retrospectiva* [33 years of the Brazilian Nursing Congress: Retrospective]. Porto Alegre, Brazil: Editora Palloti.

Sena, T. J. (1985). Perfil do enfermeiro pesquisador [Profile of the nurse researcher]. In *Anais do IV Seminário Nacional de Pesquisa em Enfermagem* (pp. 132–137). São Paulo, Brazil: Unversidade de São Paulo.

Souza, M. F. (1985). A posição do pesquisador frente aos resultados da pesquisa em enfermagem [The researcher position facing the results of nursing research]. In *Anais do IV Seminário Nacional de Pesquisa em Enfermagem* (pp. 152–156). São Paulo, Brazil: Unversidade de São Paulo.

Souza, A. M. A. (1988). Estudo de tendências da pesquisa sobre a prática de enfermagem no Brasil: 1983–1987 [The study of tendencies of research about nursing practice in Brazil: 1983–1987]. In *Anais do V Seminário Nacional de Pesquisa em Enfermagem* (pp. 95–102). Belo Horizonte, Brazil: Unversidade Federal de Minas Gerais.

Souza, A. M. A. (1991). Pesquisa em enfermagem: Impacto e perspectiva [Nursing research: Impact and perspectives] In *Anais do VI Seminário Nacional de Pesquisa em Enfermagem* (pp. 35–40). Rio de Janeiro, Brazil: Palmar Gráfica e Editora.

Stefanelli, M. C., Fukuda, I. M. K., Rolim, M. A., & Arantes. E. C. (1987). Situação da pesquisa em enfermagem psiquiátrica no Brasil [Situation of psychiatric nursing research in Brazil]. *Revista da Escola de Enfermagem da USP, 21*, 183–195.

Stefanelli, M. C., Salzano, S. D. T., & Oguisso, T. (1990). Situação da pesquisa qualitativa em enfermagem no Brasil [Situation of qualitative nursing research in Brazil]. *Revista Paulista de Enfermagem, 9*, 50–56.

Trevizan, M. A., & Mendes, I. A. C. (1983). Sobre a expansão do conhecimento, segundo Popper [About the expansion of knowledge according to Popper]. *Revista Gaúcha de Enfermagem, 4*, 215–221.

Trevizan, M. A., & Mendes, I. A. C. (1991). Iniciação cientifica: Modalidade de incentivo a pesquisa em enfermagem [Scientific initiation: Modality to stimulate nursing researeh]. *Revista Gaúcha de Enfermagem, 12*, 33–38.

Trevizan, M. A., Mendes, I. A. C., Fávero, N., & Nacarato, C. F. (1981). Atividades da enfermeira de uma unidade de internação cirúrgica [Activities of a nurse in a surgical unit]. *Enfermagem Atual, 4*, 28–31.

Vieira, T. T. (1980). *Produção científca em enfermagem no Brasil: 1960–1979*. [Nursing scientific production in Brazil: 1960–1979]. Unpublished doctoral dissertation. Universidade Federal da Bahia, Salvador, Brazil.

Index

Contents of Previous Volumes

ORDER FORM

Save 10% on Volume 15 with this coupon.

_____Check here to order the ANNUAL REVIEW OF NURSING RESEARCH, Volume 15, 1997 at a 10% discount. You will receive an invoice requesting prepayment.

Save 10% on all future volumes with a continuation order.

_____Check here to place your continuation order for the ANNUAL REVIEW OF NURSING RESEARCH. You will receive a prepayment invoice with a 10% discount upon publication of each new volume, beginning with Volume 15, 1997. You may pay for prompt shipment or cancel with no obligation.

Name _____

Institution _____

Address _____

City/State/Zip _____

Examination copies for possible adoption are available to instructors "on approval" only. Write on institutional letterhead, noting course, level, present text, and expected enrollment (include $3.50 for postage and handling). Prices slightly higher overseas. Prices subject to change.

Mail this coupon to:
SPRINGER PUBLISHING COMPANY
536 Broadway, New York, N.Y. 10012

℠ *Springer Publishing Company*

A VIRGINIA HENDERSON READER
Excellence in Nursing

Edward J. Halloran, RN, PhD, FAAN, Editor
Foreword by Angela McBride, PhD, RN, FAAN

This book provides a sampling of Virginia Henderson's classic writings in patient care, nursing education, nursing research, and nursing's role in the larger health care system. Ms. Henderson was an early advocate of autonomy for nurses and the importance of nursing scholarship—her writings have much to say to today's nurses.

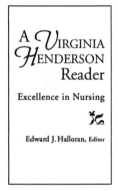

Partial Contents:

I: Patient Care. Excellence in Nursing • The Essence of Nursing in High Technology • The Art and Science of Health Assessment • The Importance of Observation

II: Nursing Education. Preparation for Specialized Nursing Graduate Programs • Nursing Process —Is the Title Right? • The Nature of Nursing • Suggestions for Basic Nursing Curricula

III: Nursing Research. Research in Nursing Practice—When? • An Overview of Nursing Research • We've "Come A Long Way" But What of the Direction? • Basis for Selection of Method: Research as a Means of Improving Nursing Practice

IV: Nursing in Society. Nursing as an Aspect of Health Care • Nursing as a Constant Factor in Health Services

1995   424pp   0-8261-8830-3   hardcover

536 Broadway, New York, NY 10012 • (212) 431-4370 • Fax (212) 941-7842